It Shouldn't Happen to a Vet

More adventures, some sad, some funny, in the life of the young vet James Herriot.

After a day of hard work in the open air, Jim can still find time to enjoy himself. He makes big plans to take out his new girlfriend – but they don't quite work out as expected! He then goes out with the wild Tristan and gets a strong taste of the local beer – but ends up on his back in the mud. Finally it is Tristan's driving, in the old Austin or in Siegfried's brand-new Rover, which nearly finishes him off.

The BULLS-EYE series

General Editor PATRICK NOBES

It Shouldn't Happen to a Vet

Adapted by Jean Nobes
from *It Shouldn't Happen to a Vet*
by James Herriot

Stanley Thornes (Publishers) Ltd

Original novel © James Herriot 1972
This adaptation © Jean Nobes 1980

Originally published in 1972 by Michael Joseph
This adaptation originally published in 1980 by Hutchinson Education
Reprinted 1981, 1982, 1984, 1986, 1988, 1989

Reprinted in 1990 by
Stanley Thornes (Publishers) Ltd
Old Station Drive
Leckhampton
CHELTENHAM GL53 0DN

British Library Cataloguing in Publication Data

Nobes, Jean
    It shouldn't happen to a vet.—(Bulls-eye book).
    1. Readers—Veterinary medicine.
    I. Title   II. Herriot, James. It shouldn't happen to a vet.
        Adaptation
    III. Series
    428'.6'2   PE1126.D4

ISBN 0 7487 0254 7

Set in Monotype Baskerville

Printed and bound in Great Britain by
The Guernsey Press Company Ltd, Guernsey, Channel Islands

Contents

1 Helping hands

Siegfried Farnon was my boss. He was the vet in Darrowby, a little market town in the Yorkshire Dales. I had worked for him for a year now. He and his brother Tristan, who was also a vet, were very interesting people to get to know. I had really enjoyed my first year, although there had been ups and downs.

Siegfried had sent me to a case that seemed simple enough. It was a case of milk fever, which sometimes happens to a cow soon after calving. The cow falls down suddenly and goes into a deep faint.

When I first saw Mr Handshaw's cow she was lying still, on her side. I had to look carefully to make sure she was not dead. The cure for milk fever is to give the cow injections of calcium, which is what they are short of. So I got out my bottles of calcium. I had been lucky enough to start work as a vet just about the time when the cure was discovered. It did not take much skill to give the shots of calcium, but it looked good.

By the time I had given her two bottles she was looking very much better. Mr Handshaw helped me to roll her on to her chest. I felt sure that, if I had the time to hang about for a bit, I would see her on her feet. However, other jobs were waiting.

'Give me a ring if she's not up by dinner time,' I said. I was pretty sure I would not have to go back again.

When the farmer rang again at mid-day to say she was still down I was not worried. Some cases needed an extra bottle. I was sure she would be all right. I went out and injected her again.

I was not really worried when she had not got up the next day, but Mr Handshaw was very upset.

'It's time the old bitch was up,' he said. 'She's doing no good lying there. Surely there's something you can do? I poured a bottle of water into her ear this morning, but even that didn't shift her.'

'You what?' I cried.

'I poured some cold water in her earhole. My dad used to get them up that way. My dad was a very clever man with cows,' he said.

'I'm sure he was,' I said, 'but I really think another injection is more likely to help her.'

As I packed up my stuff I did my best to cheer him up. I said, 'I shouldn't worry. A lot of them stay down for a day or two. Tomorrow morning she'll be walking about.'

Next day the phone rang just before breakfast. I heard Mr Handshaw's voice. It was very sad.

'She's still lying there eating her head off,' he said. 'What are you going to do now?'

What indeed, I thought as I drove out to the farm. The cow had been down for forty-eight hours. I did not like it a bit.

The farmer started in right away. 'My dad always used to say they had a worm in their tail when they stayed down like this. He said if you cut the tail off it did the trick.'

I felt bad. I had had trouble with this story before. The sad thing was that some people thought this cruel idea was true and still did it. It worked because after the tail had been cut off, the pain of the stump touching the ground made many a cow get to her feet.

'There's no such thing as a worm in the tail, Mr Handshaw,' I said. 'I hear the RSPCA man had a farmer in court last week over a job like that.'

The farmer looked at me. 'Well,' he said, 'if you won't do that, what *are* you going to do?'

I took a deep breath and said, 'Well, I'm sure she's got over the milk fever. She's eating well and she looks happy. There's no point in giving her any more calcium. I'll give her a shot of something else to try to cheer her up a bit.'

As I got the injection ready I was filled with gloom. I did not think it would work for a moment, but I had to do something.

I was just turning to go, when Mr Handshaw called after me. 'Hey! I remember something else my dad used to do. Shout in their ears. He got many a cow up that way. I'm not very strong in the voice. So how about you having a go?'

Feeling rather a fool, I went over to the cow and took hold of her ear. I took a deep breath, bent down and yelled into its hairy ear. The cow stopped chewing for a moment and looked at me. Then she went on chewing the cud.

'We'll give her another day. If she's still down to-morrow we'll have a go at lifting her. Could you get a few friends to give us a hand?' I asked.

As I expected, she was still down the next day. I got out of my car to find a group of Mr Handshaw's friends waiting for me. They were in a happy mood and full of advice. Farmers always are with somebody else's animals.

There was a lot of joking as we pushed sacks under the cow's body. Then we all gave a heave together and lifted her up. She just hung there with her legs dangling as we took her weight.

After a lot of puffing and grunting we put her down. Everybody looked at me, waiting to be told what to do. I was thinking wildly when Mr Handshaw said, 'My dad used to say a strange dog would *always* get a cow up.'

Right away there were offers of dogs. I tried to point out that one would be enough, but nobody was listening to me much any more. The men rushed home to get their dogs. It seemed only minutes before the cow-shed was full of them. The cow took no notice of them at all, except to wave her horns at them if they went too close.

The flash-point came when Mr Handshaw's own dog came in. He took one look at the strangers on his patch and then flew into action.

Within seconds the finest dog-fight I have ever seen was in full swing. The yells of the farmers rose above the growling and barking. In the middle of it all Mr Reynolds of Clover Hill was rubbing the cow's tail with two sticks and saying, 'Up! Up!'

I don't know how I heard the creaking sound over the din. Perhaps because I was bending down next to Mr Reynolds, trying to stop him rubbing the cow's tail. At that moment the cow moved a little and I heard it. The creaking came from the cow's hip or pelvis.

It took me some time to get everyone quiet again. At last they all stopped shouting and the dogs were all tied up.

'Mr Handshaw,' I asked, 'may I have a bucket of hot water, some soap and a towel, please?'

He went and got them for me, though his face showed he did not have much faith in me.

I took off my jacket, and soaped my arms. I pushed a hand into the cow's back passage. I looked up at the men and asked them to help me. I wanted two of them to get hold of the cow and rock it gently from side to side.

Yes, there it was again. I could both hear and feel it, a faint creaking.

I got up and washed my arm. I said to Mr Handshaw, 'Well, I know why your cow won't get up. She has a broken pelvis. I think she must have done it during the night she had milk fever. It's hopeless, I'm afraid.'

He looked at me and said, 'Hopeless? What do you mean?'

'I'm sorry,' I said, 'but that's how it is. The only thing you can do is get her off to a butcher. She'll never get up again.'

2 Laughing stock

That was when Mr Handshaw really blew his top. He was not rude, but he firmly told me what he thought of me as a vet. He also told me how sad it was that his dad was not here to put everything right. The other farmers stood, wide-eyed, enjoying every word.

At the end I took myself off. There was nothing more I could do. Anyway, he would have to come round to my way of thinking. Time would prove me right.

I thought of that cow as soon as I woke next morning. I was surprised when I heard Mr Handshaw's voice on the phone. I had thought it would be two or three days before he admitted he was wrong.

'Is that Mr Herriot? I'm just ringing to tell you that that cow's up on her legs and doing fine.'

'But ... but ...' was all I could say.

'Ah, you're wondering how I did it? Well, I remembered a trick of my old dad's. I went round to the butcher and got a fresh-killed sheep-skin. I put it on her back and had her up in no time. Wonderful man was my dad.'

Blindly I made my way into the dining-room. I had to talk to Siegfried about this. He listened to me as he finished his breakfast. He poured himself a last cup of coffee and said,

'Hard luck, James. The old sheep-skin trick, eh? Funny, you've been in the Dales over a year now and never come across that one, You know, like all these old cures, it has some sense in it. There's a lot of heat in a fresh sheep-skin. Very hot for a while on the back. If a cow is lying down just to be obstinate she'll get up just to get rid of it.'

I thought for a moment and said, 'But, dammit, how about the broken pelvis? It was creaking and wobbling all over the place!'

'Well, James,' said Siegfried, 'you're not the first to be caught that way. Sometimes the pelvis stays loose for a few days after calving.'

'Oh, God,' I moaned, 'what a stupid mess I've made of the whole thing!'

'Not really,' said Siegfried, as he lit a cigarette. 'That old cow was probably thinking of getting up just when she had the sheep-skin put on her. Don't you remember what I told you when you came here? One day you look a very fine vet; the next day you look a real fool. It happens to us all the time. Forget about it, James.'

To forget was not so easy, though. The cow became famous. Whenever Mr Handshaw showed her to people he said, 'That's the cow Mr Herriot said would never walk again.'

3   A friend for Tricki Woo

Siegfried put down the phone. I could not tell from
his face what he was thinking. He said, 'That was
Mrs Pumfrey. She wants you to see her pig.'

'Peke, you mean,' I said.

'No, pig. She wants you to check over her six-week-
old pig,' said Siegfried.

I laughed and said, 'All right, all right, don't start
again. What did she really want? Is Tricki Woo's
bottom playing up again?'

'James,' said Siegfried, 'it's not like you to think
I'm lying. Mrs Pumfrey told me that she's just bought
a six-week-old pig. She wants you to have a look at it
to make sure it's healthy. I want you to make a good
job of it. Now get a move on.'

I felt very puzzled as I made my way to the car. I
was used to a bit of leg-pulling since I became Tricki
the Peke's uncle.* So I really thought Siegfried must
be joking about a pig. The idea of Mrs Pumfrey with
a pig was stupid. There was no room for pigs in her
splendid house.

But he *had* been telling the truth. Mrs Pumfrey
met me with a joyful cry.

'Oh, Mr Herriot, isn't it wonderful? I have the most
darling little pig. I was staying with some friends who
are farmers and I picked him out. He will be such company for Tricki. You know how I worry about him
being an only dog.'

'You mean you really have this pig in the house?' I
asked.

*See *If Only They Could Talk*, also a Bulls-Eye book.

'Of course,' said Mrs Pumfrey. She looked surprised. 'He's in the kitchen. Come and see him.'

Mrs Pumfrey's kitchen was shining clean. Everything was as spotless as a lab. A box stood in one corner. I saw a tiny pig in it. He stood on his hind legs with his front legs on the edge of the box. He looked very happy.

'Isn't he sweet?' said Mrs Pumfrey as she tickled the little head. 'It's such fun having a pig of my own! I am going to call him Nugent.'

'Nugent?' I asked.

'Yes, Nugent. After my great uncle Nugent. He was a little pink man with tiny eyes and a little snub nose. My piggy looks very much like him.'

'I see,' I said. I really did not know what else to say.

'Come now, Nugent. Be a good boy and let your Uncle Herriot look at you.'

I picked Nugent up by his tail and took his temperature. I then sounded his heart and lungs. I looked into his eyes, ran my fingers over his limbs and checked his joints.

I felt rather a cheat as I did this, because I could see at a glance he was a very healthy little animal. However, I had found that being Tricki's uncle was a very good thing. It was not just the presents that came very often. It was also the sherry before lunch and the comfort of Mrs Pumfrey's splendid house. I enjoyed being Tricki's uncle. The way I saw it, if I was going to be Nugent's uncle too, why should I worry?

When I had finished checking the little pig over, I said to Mrs Pumfrey, 'Sound in wind and limb. You've got a very fine pig here, but there's just one thing. He can't live in the house.'

4 False alarm

Mrs Pumfrey was upset at the idea at first. But when I told her that he would not die of cold and would, in fact, be happier out-side, she gave way.

So Nugent had a beautiful sty built for him in a corner of the garden. His trough was filled twice a day with the best meal and he was never short of an extra treat like a carrot or some cabbage. Every day he was let out to play and he spent a happy hour running round the garden with Tricki.

In short, Nugent had it made. However, he was a very nice pig. He liked people. I often saw him taking a stroll round the garden with Mrs Pumfrey.

Pigs grow quickly and he soon left the pink baby stage, but was still full of charm. More than anything else, he loved having his back scratched.

There is one thing about Nugent I shall always remember. One day the phone rang. It was Mrs Pumfrey. I could tell from her voice she was very upset.

'Oh, Mr Herriot,' she said, 'thank heavens you are in. It's Nugent! I'm afraid he's very ill.'

'Really? I'm sorry to hear that. What's he doing?' I asked.

For a moment she did not say anything, then she spoke again. 'Well, he can't manage . . . well . . . not in the right way.'

'That's strange,' I said. 'Is he eating all right?'

'I think so, but . . . something is . . . stopping it. You will come, won't you?' she said.

'I'm on my way,' I said.

I had quite a long wait out-side Nugent's run. He thought I had come to play with him. When he grew bored with waiting he trotted up and down the run a few times. Mrs Pumfrey pointed a shaking finger at him.

'Oh, God,' she said. 'There! There! There it is now!' She had gone very pale.

I watched Nugent very closely. He had stopped running about and he was passing water happily. The normal male pig does this in spurts, and not in one long stream.

'I really can't see anything wrong there,' I said to Mrs Pumfrey.

'But he's doing it . . . in fits and starts!' she said.

There had been plenty of time for me to learn how to keep a straight face when talking to Mrs Pumfrey.

'But they all do that, Mrs Pumfrey,' I said.

She looked at me and said, 'You mean . . . all boy pigs . . .?'

I told her that every male pig I had ever known had done it like that. The poor lady had gone very red. She must have felt rather silly, so I said, 'Yes, indeed. Lots of people make the same mistake. Ah, well, I'd better be on my way. It's been nice to see Nugent looking so well and happy.'

Nugent enjoyed a long and happy life and, I am pleased to say, he was just as kind as Tricki with his presents. I was really fond of him. Siegfried had pulled my leg in the past when I was given the signed photo of the dog. I never dared let him see the one of the pig!

5 Why be a vet?

My first visit, one morning, took me up on one of the
narrow roads without fences which joins two of the
Dales together. When I had driven to the top I pulled
the car on to the grass and got out. From up there
you could see over the plain of York to the hills
beyond. Behind me the moorland rolled away, dip-
ping and rising over the flat fell top. In my year at
Darrowby I must have stood here often. The view
always looked different.

Today the patch-work of fields slept in the sun. The
air was heavy with the smells of summer. There must
be people working down there, I knew, but I could
not see a living soul. I was filled with the peace which
I always found on the empty moor.

At these times I seemed to stand out-side myself. It
was easy to flick back over the years to the time when
I first decided to be a vet. I could remember the very
moment. I was 13 and I was reading a book about
careers. As I read about being a vet I was suddenly
sure that this was the life for me. Yet what was behind
my wish? Only that I liked cats and dogs and did not
want to work in an office. I knew nothing about the
land or about farm animals. Though I learnt about
these things at college I could only see one future for
me. I was going to be a *small* animal vet.

Then how on earth did I come to be sitting on a
high Yorkshire moor, smelling of cows?

The change in my outlook had come quite suddenly.
It had been almost as soon as I had come to Darrowby.
The job had been a god-send. In those days of

unemployment before the war I was glad to get any job. I thought it was only a stepping-stone to what I really wanted to do. All my ideas had changed almost in a flash. Perhaps it was something to do with the sweetness of the air. The sweet smell still surprised me every morning when I stepped out into the garden. Perhaps it was life with my boss, Siegfried, and his brother Tristan. Or it could be that I found treating cows and pigs and sheep much more interesting than I had thought.

Anyway, it had all changed for me. My work meant driving from farm to farm, across the roof of England. I felt very lucky.

6 Summer milk fever

I got back in my car and looked at my list of visits. The day passed quickly. It was about seven o'clock in the evening. I thought my work was over, but then I had a phone call. It was from Terry Watson, a young farmer who kept two cows of his own. One of them, he said, had summer milk fever. In the summer months we saw hundreds of these cases. A lot of farmers called it 'August Bag'. It was a nasty thing because we never seemed to be able to cure it. Usually the cow lost part of its udder, and sometimes its life.

Terry Watson's cow looked very sick. She had limped in from the field at milking-time. Now she stood trembling in her stall, staring straight in front of her. I drew gently at the teat that was infected. Instead of milk a stream of foul-smelling muck came out.

'Can't mistake that stink, Terry,' I said. I felt the hot, swollen part of the udder. 'It looks bad, I'm afraid.'

Terry looked grim. He was in his twenties. His wife had a small baby. He worked all day for somebody else and then came home to start work on his own stock. His two cows and a few pigs and hens helped him to live on his small wage.

'I can't understand it,' he said. 'It's usually dry cows that get it. This one still gives two gallons a day.'

'No, I'm afraid all cows can get it,' I said. I had just taken the cow's temperature. It was 106.

'What's going to happen, then? Can you do anything for her?' Terry asked.

'I'll do what I can, Terry. I'll give her an injection. You must milk that teat as often as you can to get rid of that muck. But you know as well as I do that it's a poor outlook with these jobs.'

'Yes, I know all about it,' he said, watching me give the cow an injection. 'She'll lose that part of her udder, won't she? And maybe she'll even die.'

I tried to be cheerful. 'Well, I don't think she'll die. Even if she loses one-quarter of her udder she'll make it up on the other three.' But I felt helpless. I always did when I could not do much about something that really mattered.

'Look, is there nothing I can do myself?' Terry Watson asked. His thin cheeks were pale. I looked at him and thought, not for the first time, that he did not look strong enough for this hard trade.

I said, 'The cases that do best are the ones that have the most work put into them. The more you milk that teat, the more chance she has. So work away at it this evening. Every half-an-hour, if you can manage it. That rubbish in her quarter can't do any harm if you draw it out as soon as it is formed. And I think you ought to bathe the udder and massage it well.'

'What shall I rub it with?' he asked. 'I've got a bowl of goose grease.' I told him to use that.

Terry seemed glad of the chance of doing something. He got an old bucket and sat down on the milking stool.

He looked up at me and said, 'Right, I'm starting now.'

As it happened I was called out early next morning. On the way home I looked in on the Watsons' house. The time was about eight o'clock. When I went into the little shed, Terry was sitting in the same place I had left him the night before. He was pulling at the infected teat, eyes closed, head resting against the cow's side.

He looked round when I said, 'Hello, you're having another go, I see.'

The cow turned to look at me when I spoke. I saw right away that she was much better. She had lost her blank stare and she was chewing the cud.

'My God, Terry! She looks a lot better. She isn't the same cow!'

Terry was having a job keeping his eyes open, but he smiled and said, 'Yes, and come and look at this end.'

I bent down by the udder. I felt for the painful swelling of the night before. I could not believe it. The swelling had gone, and the cow seemed fine. I drew on the teat. Out came a stream of pure white milk.

'What's going on here, Terry? You must have changed cows. You're having me on, aren't you?' I asked.

'No, Mr Herriot,' said Terry with a smile. 'It's the same cow, all right. She's better, that's all.'

'But it's impossible! What the devil have you done to her?'

'Just what you told me to do,' he answered. I

scratched my head and said, 'But she's fine. I've never seen anything like it.'

'I know you haven't,' said a woman's voice from the door. I turned to see that Mrs Watson had come into the shed. She went on, 'You've never met a man who would work on a cow round the clock, have you? He's been on that stool since you left him last night. Never to bed, never been in to have a meal. Great fool. It's enough to kill anybody.'

I looked at Terry, then at the nearly empty bowl of goose grease at his feet. 'Good Lord, man,' I said. 'You must be all in. Anyway the cow's as good as new. You don't need to do another thing to her. You can go in and have a bit of a rest,' I said to Terry.

He shook his head and said, 'No, I can't do that. I've got my work to go to, and I'm late as it is.'

There was work to be done and Terry went out to get on with it.

7 Siegfried butts in

I don't know why, but I was always nervous when Siegfried watched me doing anything. I always started to go to pieces as soon as I felt him near me. I could feel that he did not like the way I did things. Not that I could tell by his face. His face did not show what he was thinking. I felt that I was not doing things the way he would do them, or I was not working fast enough, or I was doing something stupid.

One day I had just opened up a big dog that had swallowed a ball. I had found the ball, and was sewing the dog up again when Siegfried came in. I had been feeling quite happy. It had been a nice easy job that I liked doing and Tristan was helping me. Now everything was different.

Siegfried was standing quietly at the foot of the table. As the minutes passed I had the feeling that I was near a volcano that was about to explode. The explosion came when I started to stitch up the thick layer of flesh on the dog's belly. I was pulling some cat-gut out of a glass jar when I heard him catch his breath.

'God help us, James, stop pulling at that bloody cat-gut! Do you know how much it costs? Well, it's a good job you don't, or you would faint. And that dusting powder you're chucking about costs the earth. There must be half a pound inside the dog already,' he said. 'Another thing, a small bit of cotton-wool is enough for a swab. You don't need a square foot at a time like you've been using. Here, give me the needle. I'll show you!'

He quickly scrubbed his hands and took over. First he took a tiny pinch of the dusting powder and sprinkled it into the wound. It was rather like watching an old lady feeding her goldfish. Then he cut off a little bit of gut and began to sew up the wound. He had hardly left himself enough to tie the knot at the end. It was touch and go, but he just made it.

'Right, turn off the gas, Tristan,' he said, turning to his brother. Siegfried pulled off half an inch of cotton-wool and wiped the wound down.

He turned to me and smiled. He said, 'James, don't get the wrong end of the stick. You've made a grand job of this dog, but you've got to keep one eye on cost. I know it doesn't matter a hoot to you at the moment, but some day you'll be your own boss. Then you'll know some of the worries I have on my shoulders.' He patted my arm and went on, 'After all,

James, you'll agree we ought to make some profit in the end.'

I managed not to say a word, but I felt cross.

8 Horse-play

It was a week later and I was helping Siegfried with an operation on a horse. I was giving the horse the anaesthetic, something I often did. Siegfried was a splendid horse doctor, far better than me, so I always gave the anaesthetic and he did the rest of the work.

We liked to do the operations in the open, which was cleaner than indoors. Also, if the horse was wild there was less chance of him hurting himself. We always hoped for a fine morning and that day we were lucky.

Everything had gone more or less as usual. I had gone into the box with the horse, put on the muzzle, and walked him out to the field. There, as a man walked him slowly round, I gave him some anaesthetic on a sponge. I kept adding a little more each time, till the horse began to stagger and sway. This stage always took a few minutes. Then the horse gave a final stagger and went down on his side.

Siegfried sprang into action. 'Sit on his head!' he yelled. 'Get a rope on that upper hind leg and pull it forward! Bring me that bucket of water! Come on, move!'

That morning's case was an injury. A bad one, needing an anaesthetic for the operation. The horse had been galloping round his paddock and suddenly decided to escape. He had chosen the only sharp fence to try to jump over, and had been caught on it. In his efforts to get away he had cut the flesh on his chest, which looked like something from the butcher's shop. The skin was cut and the flesh was hanging.

'Roll him on his back,' said Siegfried. 'That's better.'

He took a probe and looked at the wound very carefully.

'No damage to the bone,' he said. Then he used the probe to fish out all the loose dirt he could find. Then he turned to me and said, 'It's just a big stitching job. You can carry on if you like.'

We changed places. As I picked up the needle I suddenly remembered opening up that dog. Maybe I was on trial for my wasteful ways. This time I would be careful.

I took a very tiny bit of cat-gut and began to sew everything back into place. Using little short ends of gut was a slow way of doing the job and I took about three times longer than usual. However, I kept going.

I had put in about six stitches this way when I felt the waves of anger coming from Siegfried. I kept going for another two stitches when he exploded. He hissed at me, so nobody could hear, 'What the hell are you playing at, James?'

I was surprised so I said, 'Just stitching. What do you mean?'

'Why are you messing about with all those little bits of gut? We'll be here all day!' Siegfried said, and swore at me.

'I'm using little bits of gut so that I don't waste any,' I said, going on with my work.

'I can't stand any more of this! Here, let me have a go,' said Siegfried.

He picked up a needle. Then he caught hold of the end of the cat-gut that was sticking out of the jar. He pulled out a very long piece of gut and began to stitch. The gut was so long that he had to stretch his arm to pull every stitch tight. In spite of this he finished sewing the inside stitches in record time.

He spotted a drop of blood coming from somewhere. He tore off a mass of cotton-wool from the roll and wiped the blood away.

'Just a touch of powder before I stitch the out-side skin,' he said. He grabbed the box of powder and waved it around over the horse. Some of the powder went into the wound, but much more went over the rest of the horse, me and the grass.

Siegfried finished the job, using several yards of silk. He looked at the tidy result and was pleased with himself.

'Well now, that's fine,' he said. 'I don't think it will leave a mark.' He came over and talked to me as I washed the instruments.

'Sorry I pushed you out like that, James. Quite honestly I couldn't think what had come over you. You were like an old hen. It looks bad, trying to work with tiny bits of stuff. If you stint yourself you don't look as if you're really sure what you're doing.'

I finished washing the instruments, dried them and put them away. Then I started to walk across the field. As we walked, Siegfried put his hand on my shoulder, and said, 'Mind you, don't think I'm blaming you, James. I suppose it's because you're Scottish. I'm sure you'll admit that you Scots some-times stint yourselves too much for the sake of a few pence.'

I felt like hitting him.

He went on, 'I know I don't have to keep on at you, James. You always take notice of what I say, don't you?'

'Yes,' I said, 'I do. Every single time!'

9 Pig-talk

'I can see you like pigs,' said Mr Worley as I was getting into his pig pen.

I asked him how he knew.

He said, 'Oh, I can always tell. You went in there nice and quiet, and scratched Queenie's back and spoke to her. I said to myself, "there's a young man who likes pigs".'

'Well, as a matter of fact I do like pigs,' I said. I had really been creeping past Queenie, wondering what she would do. She was a huge sow. Sows with a litter of piglets can be very stroppy with strangers. When I went into the building she had got up from where she was feeding her piglets and given me a very funny look. It made me think of the number of times I had left a pig pen a lot quicker than I went in. A big, angry sow has always been able to make me move very fast.

Now I was right in the pen and Queenie did not seem to mind me. She lay down and went on feeding her family. Now I could have a look at her foot, which was why I had come.

'Yes, that's the one,' said Mr Worley. 'She could hardly walk this morning.'

There did not seem to be much wrong. A flap of the horn of one claw was a bit over-grown. It was rubbing on the sole of the foot. We did not usually get called out for little things like that. I cut away the over-grown bit and put some ointment on. All the time Mr Worley knelt by Queenie's head, patted her and spoke in her ear. I could not make out the words he used. Perhaps it was pig-talk, because the sow talked back to him in little grunts. Anyway, it worked better than an anaesthetic. Everyone was happy, even the little piglets, working away at the two rows of teats.

When I had finished I gave Mr Worley the ointment, telling him to rub it into the foot twice a day.

'Thank you, I'm very grateful,' he said. He shook my hand as if I had saved the pig's life. 'I'm very glad to meet you for the first time, Mr Herriot. I've known Mr Farnon for a long time and I think very highly of him. He loves pigs, that man. His young brother has been here once or twice. I think he's fond of pigs, too.'

I told him I was sure Tristan loved pigs. He smiled and said, 'Yes, I thought so. I can always tell.'

We went out into what was really the back yard of a pub. Mr Worley was not a full-time farmer, he was the landlord of the pub as well. His pigs were in what had once been the stables.

For years expert farmers had been telling Mr Worley that he would never do any good with his pigs. If you were going in for breeding, they said, you had to have a proper pig-house. It was not a bit of good putting your sows into make-shift pens like his. For years Mr Worley's sows had given him big litters, and looked after them with loving care. They were all good mothers and did not hurt their families or crush them by accident. Over and over again at the end of eight weeks he had twelve healthy pigs to take to market. None of the expert farmers did as well as that.

As I came to know Mr Worley better I found that pigs mattered to him more than anything else. Knowing him better had its own rewards. The time I feel most like a glass of beer is not in the evening when the pubs are open. It's around 4.30 on a hot summer afternoon after I've been working hard. It was lovely to sit in Mr Worley's back kitchen and sip at the cool bitter ale straight from the cellar below.

Mostly we were on our own. When Mr Worley had brought the tall jug up from the cellar he would sit down and say, 'Well, let's have a piggy talk!'

He seemed to love our long talks on anything and everything to do with pigs. Once, in the middle of a chat about how many windows a pig-house should have, he stopped suddenly. He blinked behind his glasses and burst out, 'You know, Mr Herriot, sitting here like this with you, I'm as happy as a king.'

10   Marigold

I was often called out for very small problems because of Mr Worley's fondness for his pigs. I swore under my breath when I heard his voice on the other end of the phone at one o'clock one morning. 'Marigold pigged this afternoon, Mr Herriot. I don't think she's got much milk. The little pigs look hungry to me. Will you come?' he asked.

I got out of bed, went downstairs and through the long garden to the yard. By the time I had got the car out into the lane I had begun to wake up. When I rolled up to the pub I was able to greet Mr Worley fairly cheerfully.

But the poor man did not smile. In the light from the oil lamp he was grey with worry. 'I hope you can do something quickly,' he said. 'I'm really upset about her. She's just lying there doing nothing. It's such a lovely litter, too. Fourteen she's had.'

I could see why he was worried as I looked in the pen. Marigold lay still on her side. The tiny piglets rushed from teat to teat, squealing and falling over each other in a wild hunt for food. Their little bodies had a thin, empty look. This meant their bellies were empty. I hated to see a litter starve to death, but it could happen so easily. There came a time when they stopped trying to suck and began to lie about the pen. After that it was hopeless.

I asked if the sow had eaten the evening before, and Mr Worley said she had eaten as usual. I took her temperature. It was normal. I ran my hands along the udder, pulling in turn at the teats. The udder seemed full, but I could not get even a drop of milk out.

'There's nothing there, is there?' asked Mr Worley sadly.

I turned to him and said, 'There's no milk fever, and Marigold isn't really ill. But there is something stopping her giving milk. She's got plenty of milk, so I'll give her an injection of something to help her let it down.'

I tried not to look pleased as I spoke, because this was one of my best party tricks. There is something that looks like magic in the injection vets use in these cases. It works within a minute and it does not need any skill. The result is marvellous.

I gave the injection. I waited nearly a minute, then I reached down again to the udder.

Mr Worley looked surprised. 'What are you doing now?' he asked.

'Having a feel to see if the milk has come down yet,' I said.

'Why, damn, it can't be!' he said. 'You've only just given her the jab!'

This was going to be good. With finger and thumb I took hold of one of the teats. I directed my shot past Mr Worley's left ear, but I got my aim wrong and sprinkled his glasses instead!

He took them off and wiped them slowly as if he could not believe what he had seen. Then he bent over and tried for himself. 'It's a miracle!' he cried as the milk splashed over his hand. 'I've never seen anything like it!'

It did not take the little pigs long to catch on. Within a few seconds they had stopped fighting and squealing and settled down in a long silent row. They were going to make up for lost time.

I went into the kitchen to wash my hands. I was drying them on the towel behind the door when I heard something odd. I heard people talking. It seemed strange in a pub at two o'clock in the morning. I looked through the half open door into the bar. The place was crowded. I could see a row of men drinking at the counter, while others sat behind pints on the seats against the walls.

Mr Worley grinned and said, 'You didn't expect to see this lot, did you? Well, the real drinkers don't come in till after closing time. Every night I lock the front door and these lads come round the back.'

I pushed my head round the door for another look. All the criminals in the town were there. Then they saw me, and cries of welcome rang out. Above the rest a voice said, 'Are you going to have a drink?' What I wanted most was to get back to bed, but it would look bad just to shut the door and go. I went in and over to the bar. I seemed to have plenty of friends there. In seconds I was in the middle of a merry group with a pint in my hand.

Then I saw that the men were looking at me as if they were waiting for something. So was the girl behind the bar.

'Six pints of best bitter. Six shillings, please,' she said.

I took the money out of my pocket. It seemed I was wrong in thinking somebody had asked me to have a drink. I finished my beer and left as soon as I could.

I could see the light from the pig pen as I crossed the yard. Mr Worley was still talking to his sow. He looked up as I came in. His face was shining with happiness.

'Mr Herriot,' he said, 'isn't that a beautiful sight?'

He pointed to the little pigs. They were lying on each other, sound asleep, bellies fat with Marigold's milk.

'It is indeed,' I said. 'You would have to go a long way to beat it.'

I really *was* pleased too. As I got into the car I felt that the visit had been worth-while – even if I had been tricked into buying a round.

As luck would have it Mr Worley's pub was raided that night. A police-man had come by on his bike ten minutes after I had left and caught everybody in the place.

Mr Worley was fined £15 but I don't think he really minded. Marigold and her litter were doing well.

11 A runaway

At one time Tristan was driving me around, because I had my arm in a sling. It had been infected after a bad calving. Every time we came to a gate I had to jump out of the car and open it.

This was the last gate. I got out to open it, and looked back at the farm. It was a long way below us now. Some of these Dales farms were strange places. This one had no road to it, not even a track. You drove across the fields from gate to gate until you reached the main road above the valley.

Tristan did not drive through the gate. He got out of the car, leaned his back against the gate post and lit a cigarette. He was not in a hurry. With a happy smile he shut his eyes. The sun was warm on the back of his neck and his stomach was full of beer that the farmer had given us at the farm down in the valley. I could see he felt pretty good.

He opened his eyes quickly as a creaking noise came from the car. 'Hell! She's off, Jim!' he shouted.

The little Austin was moving gently back down the slope. It must have slipped out of gear, and it had no brakes to speak of. We both ran after it. Tristan just managed to touch the bonnet with one finger, but he could not keep up with the car. The speed was too much for us. We gave up the chase and watched.

The hill-side was steep, and the little car bounced crazily over the uneven ground. I looked at Tristan. I had a good idea what he was thinking. It was only two weeks since he had turned the Hillman over, taking a girl home from a dance. It had been a write-off. The insurance people had been quite nasty about it. Of course, Siegfried had gone nearly mad. He had sacked Tristan once and for all, he never wanted to see his face again.

But Tristan had been sacked very often. He knew he had only to keep out of his brother's way for a bit. Siegfried would soon forget. Tristan had been lucky because Siegfried had talked his bank manager into letting him buy a beautiful new Rover. This had put everything else out of his mind.

The Austin seemed to be doing about seventy miles an hour, bumping down the long green hill. One by one the doors burst open. Soon all four were flapping wildly as the car ran down the hill.

From the open doors bottles, instruments, bandages and cotton-wool fell out on to the grass.

Tristan threw up his arms and cried, 'Look! The damn thing is going straight for that hut!'

Indeed, the hut was the only thing on the hill, and the Austin was rushing straight towards it.

I could not bear to watch. I turned away. When the crash came I looked back down the hill. The hut was gone. On top of the broken planks the little car lay on its side, its wheels still turning.

As we went down the hill it was easy to guess Tristan's thoughts. He would not be looking forward to telling Siegfried about the Austin. When we got to the car we had a good look at it. We could not make out whether there were any new marks on the body, as it had been so bashed and dented before. The rear end was a bit smashed in, but this did not show up much. The only other new damage seemed to be a broken rear light. Our hopes rising we set off to the farm for help.

The farmer seemed pleased to see us again. 'Now then, you lads,' he said, 'have you come back for some more beer?'

'That's a nice idea,' said Tristan, 'but we've had a bit of an accident.'

We went into the house and the kind man opened some more bottles. He did not seem worried when he heard what had happened to the hut.

'No, that's not mine. Belongs to the golf club. It's the club-house,' he said.

Tristan's eye-brows shot up. 'Oh no! Don't say we've smashed the head-quarters of the Darrowby golf club!'

'You must have,' said the farmer. 'It's the only wooden hut in those fields. I rent that part of my land to the club. They've made a little nine-hole golf course. Don't worry, hardly anybody plays on it. Only the bank manager, and I don't like the fellow.'

The farmer lent us a horse and we went back to the car and pulled it upright again.

Trembling a little, Tristan pressed the car's starter. The sturdy little engine burst into a roar straight away. He drove carefully over the broken hut on to the grass.

Tristan thanked the farmer for the loan of his horse, and said, 'We seem to have got away with it.'

The farmer smiled and said, 'Your car is as good as new.' Then he winked and added, 'Now, you say nothing about this job and I'll say nothing. Right?'

'Right! Come on, Jim, get in.' Tristan put his foot down and we chugged up the hill once more.

12   Tristan gets lucky

Tristan did not speak until we reached the road. Then he turned to me and said, 'You know, Jim, I've still got to tell Siegfried about that rear light. Don't you think it's a bit hard the way I get blamed for everything that happens to his cars? You've seen it over and over again. He gives me a lot of old wrecks to drive. When they start to fall to bits, it's always my fault. It isn't fair.'

'Well, Siegfried isn't the man to suffer in silence,' I said. 'He's got to lash out, and you're nearest.'

Tristan was silent for a moment, then he said, 'Mind you, I'm not saying it wasn't my fault that the Hillman was a write-off. I was taking that sharp turn at sixty, with my arm round a nurse. But all in all, I've had very bad luck.'

Siegfried was out of sorts when he got back home. He was starting a summer cold and was not feeling well, but he was hopping mad at the news.

'You madman!' he shouted. 'God help me, I think all I work for is to pay the bills that you run up. Go on, get the hell out of here! I'm finished with you.'

Tristan did what he usually did at these times and lay low. He did not see his brother until the next morning. Siegfried was feeling worse. His cold had given him a sore throat, and he had lost his voice. When Tristan and I went into his bed-room he was reading the local paper.

He spoke to us in a whisper. 'Have you seen this? It says here that the golf club-house was knocked down yesterday. No clue how it happened. Damn funny thing!' His head lifted suddenly from the pillow and he glared at Tristan. 'You were at that farm yesterday!' He fell back muttering. 'Oh, no, no. I'm sorry. It's too silly. It's wrong of me to blame you for everything.'

Tristan looked worried. He had never heard this kind of talk from Siegfried before. I was worried too. Could my boss be really ill?

'I've just had a call from Mr Armitage at Sorton,' said Siegfried, finding it hard to speak. 'He's got a cow down with milk fever. I want you to drive James out there straight away. Go on, now. Get moving.'

'I'm afraid I can't,' Tristan said. 'Jim's car is in the garage. They're fixing that light. It'll take them about an hour.'

'Well, Armitage is in a bit of a panic. That cow could be dead in an hour. What the hell can we do?' Siegfried said.

'There's the Rover,' said Tristan.

Terror showed in Siegfried's eyes. With an effort he pulled himself on to his side and stared into his brother's eyes. He hissed slowly at Tristan, 'Right, so you'll have to take the Rover. Just let me tell you this. If you put a scratch on that car, I'll kill you. I'll kill you with my own two hands.'

Tristan did not say a word. I followed him out of the bed-room. I glanced back as I was going through the door. Siegfried looked as if he was praying.

Out-side the room Tristan rubbed his hands together.

'What a break, Jim!' he said. 'You know, I never thought I'd get behind the wheel of that Rover for a hundred years. Just shows you, everything happens for the best!'

13 A lucky escape

Five minutes later he was backing out of the yard and into the lane. Once on the Sorton road I saw he was beginning to enjoy himself. For two miles the road ahead stretched straight and clear. A long way off there was a milk lorry coming towards us. A perfect place to see what the Rover could do. Tristan pressed his foot down hard.

We were doing eighty when I saw a car start to over-take the milk lorry. I waited for it to pull back but it still came on. The driver of the milk lorry seemed to have decided to make a race of it and put on speed.

With alarm I saw the two of them abreast and coming towards us. They were only a few hundred yards away, and not a foot of space on either side of them. Tristan put on his brakes. If the lorry did the same the car would just be able to squeeze between us. But within seconds I saw that the lorry was not braking. We were bound to crash.

I closed my eyes. Then something hit the side of the

Rover. When I opened my eyes our car had stopped. We were sitting there, staring ahead at the empty road.

I listened to the thumping of my heart. Then I looked back to see the lorry nearly out of sight round a distant bend. I noticed that Tristan's face was really green. I had never seen a green face before.

I could feel the wind coming in from the left. There were no doors on that side. One lay by the road-side a few yards back, the other hung from a single broken hinge. Slowly, as if in a dream, I got out and looked at the damage. The left side of the Rover was a mess of twisted metal.

Tristan sat down on the grass, his face blank. This state did not last long. He began to blink and to look for his cigarettes. What was he going to do now?

It seemed to me there were only three things he could do. First, he could get out of Darrowby and go abroad if possible. Second, he could get on the first train out of Darrowby, and go home to mother until all this had blown over. Third, and I could hardly bear to think about it, he could tell Siegfried he had smashed up his new Rover.

As I thought things over I spotted the old car that had hit us. It was lying upside down in a ditch about fifty yards down the road. As we hurried towards it I heard a lot of noise coming from inside. I remembered that it was market day in Darrowby. Farmers would be bringing crates of hens and twenty or thirty dozen eggs to sell.

We looked in through the window and gasped. A fat man, unhurt, was lying in a great pool of smashed eggs. There was a wide smile on the part of his face we could see through the eggs. The rest of the inside of the car was filled with noisy hens.

The fat man, smiling up happily from his bed of eggs, was shouting something. It was hard to hear him above the noise of the hens. I caught snatches of what he was saying.

'Very sorry indeed – all my fault – I'll make good the damage.'

'Are you all right?' Tristan shouted, opening the door.

'Yes, yes, young man, I'm not hurt. Please don't worry about me. I'm sorry about this, but I'll see you're all right, you can be sure.'

He held out a dripping hand and we helped him out on to the road.

'You know what the trouble was, don't you?' he said to Tristan. 'The sun got in my eyes.'

It was twelve noon so the sun shone directly above, and the man had been driving north, but there did not seem any point in saying anything.

We put the damaged doors back inside the Rover, drove to Sorton, treated the milk fever and went back to Darrowby. Tristan gave me a scared look, then marched straight to his brother's room. I went after him.

Siegfried was worse. His face was red with fever, and his eyes burned. He did not move when Tristan walked over to the foot of the bed. He said, 'Well, how did you get on?'

'Fine. The cow was on her feet when we left. There's just one thing. I had a bump with the car,' said Tristan.

Siegfried stopped breathing. Then he managed to whisper, 'What happened?'

'It wasn't my fault,' Tristan said. 'A chap tried to over-take a lorry and didn't make it. He caught one side of the Rover.'

Again the silence and again the whisper.

'Much damage?'

'Both doors torn off the left side. Not much left of the front and rear wings,' said Tristan.

Siegfried came bolt upright in bed. His mouth

opened in a soundless scream. 'You bloody fool! You're sacked!'

He crashed back on the pillow and lay very still. We watched him for a few moments in some fear. When we heard him breathing again we left the room on tip-toe.

On the landing Tristan lit a cigarette and said to me, 'That was a tricky one, Jim. But you know what I always say. Things usually turn out better than you think.'

14 A new face

One morning I was pleased to find the farm I was looking for so easily. There on its gate was written 'Heston Grange'. Often the Dales farmers did not bother to put a sign on their gates.

I got out of the car and undid the latch. The farm-house lay below me, a large, grey stone building.

I walked round the out-buildings, shouting as I always did. Some farmers did not like it if I called at the farm-house for them. Good farmers are indoors only at meal-times. But nobody answered my shouts, so I went and knocked at the door.

I was told to come in. I opened the door into the kitchen. A girl with dark hair and a check blouse and slacks was at the table making bread. She looked up and smiled. 'Sorry I couldn't let you in,' she said. 'I've got my hands full.' She held up her arms, white with flour to the elbow.

'That's all right,' I said. 'My name is James

Herriot. I've come to see a calf. It's lame, I understand.'

'Yes, we think he's broken his leg. If you don't mind waiting a minute, I'll come with you. My father and the men are in the fields. I'm Helen Alderson.'

She washed and dried her arms and put on some rubber boots. Out-side, she laughed and said to me, 'We've got a bit of a walk, I'm afraid. He's in one of the top buildings. Look, you can see it up there.' She pointed to a stone barn, high on the fell-side. I got a lot of walking done, going round these top buildings, in my job. They were used for storing hay and to shelter animals.

I looked at the girl for a few seconds, and then said, 'Oh, that's all right, I don't mind. I don't mind at all.'

We went over the field and crossed a little bridge over the river. I thought to myself that this new fashion of women wearing slacks had quite a lot to be said for it. We walked for ten minutes through a pine wood, where it was cool and silent.

Then we were out again in the hot sun on the open moor. Here the path was steeper still. I was beginning to puff, but the girl kept up a brisk pace. I was glad when we got to the level ground on the top. The barn came into sight again.

The calf looked very small and sorry for himself. One of his front legs trailed along the floor as he tried to walk. I asked the girl to hold him while I looked at him. She caught him like an expert, one hand under his chin, the other holding an ear.

I said to her, 'You were quite right. It's a clean break, so it should do well with a plaster on it.' I set to work and put a plaster on the leg. After I had finished I said, 'We'll just wait a couple of minutes, then we can let him go.' I kept tapping the plaster till I was sure it was set like stone. 'All right,' I said, 'he can go now.'

The girl let go of his head and he trotted away. 'Look!' she said. 'He's putting his weight on it already!'

I smiled. I felt I had really done something. The calf felt no pain now that he could not move the broken ends of the bone. The fear that always saddens a hurt animal had gone. 'Yes,' I said, 'he's perked up very quickly.'

I began to pack my bags, and said, 'He'll have to keep the plaster on for a month. If you give me a ring I'll come and take it off. Just keep an eye on him. Make sure his leg doesn't get sore round the top of the plaster.'

As we left the barn the sunshine and the sweet warm air met us like a wave. I looked across the valley to the green heights beyond. Beneath my feet the grass slopes fell away to where the river shone among the trees.

We sat down on the warm grass of the hill-side.

'It's wonderful up here,' I said. 'You're lucky to live here, but I don't think you need me to tell you that.'

She looked around her slowly and said, 'No, I love this country. There's nowhere else quite like it. I'm glad you like it, too. A lot of people find it too bare and wild.'

I laughed and said, 'Yes, I know, but I feel sorry for all the vets who don't work in the Yorkshire Dales.' I began to talk about my work. Then, almost without knowing it, I was going back over my student days.

I surprised myself with my flow of talk. I did not think of myself as a chatterbox and I felt I must be boring her. But she sat quietly, nodding at times as though she understood. She laughed in all the right places.

It came to me that it was a long time since I had talked to a girl. I had almost forgotten what it was like.

41

I did not hurry down the path and through the wood, but it seemed no time at all before we crossed the little bridge and walked over the fields to the farm.

As I got into the car I said, 'Well, I'll see you in a month.' It was a very long time to have to wait.

As the three of us sat eating lunch, Siegfried said, 'Helen Alderson? Of course I know her. Lovely girl.'

Tristan said nothing, but raised his eyes to the ceiling and gave a long, low whistle.

Siegfried went on again, 'Yes, I know her well. I think a lot of her. Her mother died a few years ago, and she runs the whole place. Cooks and looks after her father and younger brother and sister. Any men friends? Half the young men round here are chasing her, but she doesn't seem to be going steady with any of them. She's very fussy, I think.'

15   Money for old rope

For some time now I had been an LVI. This meant I was a Local Vet Inspector for the Ministry of Agriculture. So now I could do part-time work for the Government. I would be asked to examine cows, and also to do tests for TB. The illness was very common in those days, before we had drugs that could cure it. We knew that people caught it from drinking infected milk, so vets examined cows to check whether they had the disease. If we found it, the cow was slaughtered right away.

I soon found that the Dales farmers' idea of time was different from mine when there was TB testing to be done.

It was all right when I called on them to see a sick animal. They were usually around waiting for me, and the animal would be ready for me to look at. But it was not the same when I sent them a card saying I was coming to inspect their dairy cows or test their herd.

The card said clearly what time I was coming, and that the cows had to be indoors. I planned my day expecting to take a quarter of an hour for each examination and anything up to several hours if I had to test a big herd. If I was kept waiting for ten minutes at every examination while they got the cows in from the field, it meant that after six examinations I was running an hour late.

So when I drove up to Mr Kay's farm to do a TB test I was very pleased to find his cows ready and tied up in their stalls. We went through them in no time at all. I thought I was having a wonderful start to the day. Mr Kay said he had only another half dozen young cows for me to test, after which the job would be finished. It was when I left the buildings and saw the group of young cows grazing at the far end of a big field that my heart sank.

'I thought you'd have them all inside, Mr Kay,' I said.

'No, no,' he said, puffing away at his pipe. 'I didn't like to put them in on a grand hot day like this. We'll drive them up to that little barn at the top of the field. It won't take many minutes.'

At these last words my heart sank. I had heard those awful words so many times before. But perhaps it would be all right this time. We made our way to the bottom of the field and got behind the cows.

'Cush! Cush!' cried Mr Kay.

'Cush! Cush!' I added, clapping my hands.

The cows stopped grazing and looked at us with interest. Then they began to stroll up the hill. We managed to get them to the door of the barn, but there they stopped. The leader put her head inside the barn for a moment. Then, suddenly, she dashed down the hill. The others followed, even though we danced and waved our arms about to stop them. They ran past as if we were not there. They were enjoying this new game.

We went down the hill once more. Again there was the slow stroll up to the door, and again the dash down.

It was a long steep hill. As I marched up it for the third time, the sun blazing on my back, I began to feel sorry I had put so many clothes on. The letter from the Ministry of Agriculture had said that LVIs were meant to wear proper clothing when doing tests. I had taken it to heart and put on a long oil-skin coat and rubber boots. Not the best outfit for the job in hand. Sweat was running into my eyes and my shirt was stuck to me.

When, for the third time, I saw the cows running away from us down the hill, I said, 'Just a minute. I'm getting a bit warm.' I took off my coat and put it on the grass well away from the barn. I was wondering to myself where I had gone wrong. After all, Ministry work was easy. Any vet would tell you that. You did not have to get up in the middle of the night. You had nice set hours and it was not hard work. In fact it was money for old rope – a nice change from the real thing. I wiped my wet brow and stood panting. This was just not fair.

16 A fine trick

We tried again to get the cows into the barn, and failed again. That was our fourth try. After the eighth failure, I looked at Mr Kay. He was lighting his pipe and seemed happy enough. He did not seem to care that we had been going on like this for forty minutes.

'Look, we're getting nowhere,' I said. 'I've got a lot of other work waiting for me. Isn't there anything else we could try?'

He looked at me in mild surprise and said, 'Well, now, let's see. I think we'll have to get Sam. He'll get them in all right.'

'How's he going to do that?' I asked.

'He can make a noise like a warble fly.' He saw my look of amazement and went on, 'That's right. He's a bit slow, but one thing he can do is make a noise like a fly. I'll go and get him. He's only two fields down the road.'

As Mr Kay went off in search of Sam I lay down on the grass. Any other time I would have enjoyed lying there in the sun, but now I felt too upset. I had a full day's Ministry's work waiting for me and I was an hour behind time already. I could picture a long line of farmers waiting for me in very bad tempers. At last I saw Mr Kay coming back along the road.

Just behind him a big, fat man was riding on a very small bike. Mr Kay said, 'Sam has come to give us a hand.' I said good morning to Sam, and he turned to me and nodded. His eyes were blank. Sam did indeed look a bit slow. I did not think he would be able to help us.

The cows watched with interest as we came near. They had enjoyed every minute of this morning's game and were hoping for more.

Sam made a ring of his thumb and finger and put it to his lips. He took a deep breath. Then there came a sudden angry sound, a humming and buzzing that sounded like a warble fly coming in to sting.

The effect on the cows was electric. Gone was their happy contented air. They went stiff with fear. Then as the noise grew louder they charged up the hill.

Mr Kay and I went with them yet again up to the barn. Here they formed a group and waited. Sam fixed them with a blank stare and began to make the warble fly noise again. The cows knew when they were beaten. They turned and rushed into the barn.

A few minutes later Sam had left us and I was happily dealing with the cows. I looked at the farmer and said, 'You know, that chap has a wonderful gift.'

Mr Kay smiled sadly and said, 'Yes, he can make a noise like a warble fly all right. Poor old lad, it's the only thing he's good at.'

17 Everyone agrees

As I hurried away from Mr Kay's farm to my second test, I thought how lucky I was that it was the Hugills. The four brothers and their families ran a herd of about 200 cows. I had to test the lot of them, but I knew that they would not say a word about my being late. The Hugills were quite amazingly well mannered. Any visitor to their farm was treated like a member of the royal family.

As I drove into the farm I could see everybody coming towards me with beaming faces. The brothers were in the lead. As I looked at them I thought what I always did when I saw them: I had never seen such healthy looking men. Their ages ranged from late 40s to 60. I should say their average weight would be about fifteen stone. They were not fat, just huge, solid men with bright red faces and clear eyes.

I knew what was coming. It was always the same. One of them stepped forward and said,

'How are you today, sir?'

'Very well, thank you, Mr Hugill,' I said.

'Good!' he said, and the other brothers all said, 'Good, good, good,' with big smiles.

'How is Mr Farnon?' asked the same brother.

'He's very fit, thanks,' I said.

'Good!' he said and again from behind him came, 'Good, good, good.'

He had not finished yet. Again he asked, 'And how is young Mr Farnon?'

'In really top form,' I said.

'Good!' he said, and gave a little smile. From behind him came a few laughs. They closed their eyes and their shoulders shook silently. They all knew Tristan.

We all went into the cow-shed. I looked at the long row of backs and the tails swishing at the flies. There was some work ahead here.

'Sorry I'm so late,' I said, getting out my syringe. 'I was held up at the last place. It's difficult to plan how long these tests will take.'

All four brothers replied. 'Yes, sir, you're right. It's difficult. It *is* difficult. You're right, you're right, it's difficult.' They all went on and on and on.

I began to push my way between the first two cows. It was a tight squeeze and I puffed. 'It's a bit warm in here.'

Again they all agreed with me.

'You're right, sir. Yes, it's warm. It *is* warm. You're right. It's warm. It's warm. Yes, you're right.' They all nodded their heads as if I had been very clever. As I looked at their serious faces I began to relax. I was lucky to work here. Where else but in this part of Yorkshire would I meet people like these?

We began the hard work of checking every cow. It took an awfully long time but at last we got through it all. Then I was out in the fresh air, putting my oilskin coat in the boot of the car. I looked at my watch. Three o'clock. I was nearly two hours behind my time-table.

One of the brothers said to me, 'Come in and sit down and have a cup of tea.'

'It's very kind of you, Mr Hugill, I wish I could,' I said, 'but I've got a long string of visits waiting and I don't know when I'll get round to them. I've fixed up far too many, and I had no idea how long a test would take. I really am a stupid fool.'

The brothers all said, 'Yes, you're right, sir, you're right, you're right.'

18   What a day!

I still had ten more herds to examine. I should have been at the first of them two hours before. Gripping the wheel with one hand, I used the other to pull out a chunk of Mrs Hall's ham and egg pie from my lunch packet. I began to eat it as I drove along.

I felt better when I had eaten. I did not mind so much when the farmer at the next farm greeted me with a long face.

'This isn't one o'clock!' he shouted. 'My cows have been in all afternoon. Look at the mess they've made. I'll never get the place clean again!'

I had to agree with him when I saw the muck piled up behind the cows. It was one of the problems of keeping cows in during grass time.

'I won't keep you much longer,' I said, and began to work my way down the row. I moved from cow to cow, feeling their udders for any hard lumps. Among themselves vets called this 'bag-snatching' or 'cow-punching'. It was a job that soon got boring. I found the only way to fight the boredom was to think hard about what I was there for. By finding an infected cow I might save a child's life. A number of killer diseases were common in those days.

So when I came to a cow that I did not like the look of, I said to the farmer, 'I'm going to take a milk sample from this one. She's a bit hard in the left hind quarter.'

The farmer sniffed and said, 'Please yourself. There's nothing wrong with her, but I suppose it'll make a job for somebody.'

I stuck a label on the sample bottle and put it in the car. Coming back into the cow-shed I looked carefully at the wall in front of each cow. The farmer watched me and asked what I was doing.

I said, 'Well, if a cow has a cough you can often find some spit on the wall.' In fact, I had found more cows with TB in this way than in any other.

At the next four places I visited the farmers had got tired of waiting for me, and had turned their cows out to grass. They all had to be brought in and they all came in slowly. A lot more time was lost. As I ran to and fro, each farmer told me the same thing. Cows only like to come in at milking time.

When milking time came I caught three of my herds while they were being milked. But it was after six when I came, tired and hungry, to my second to last visit. I could not find the farmer round the farm, so I asked for him at the farm-house.

His wife said, 'He's had to go into the village to get the horse shod. It won't be long before he's back. He's left the cows in for you.'

That was fine. I would soon get through this lot. I almost ran into the cow-shed and started the job. I felt sick to death of the sight and smell of cows. I was working along the line when I came to a thin cow with a red and white face. I had only just touched her udder when she kicked out and caught me just above the kneecap.

I hopped around on one leg, groaning and swearing with pain. It was some time before I was able to limp back to have another try. This time I scratched her back and talked softly before trying to touch her udder. The same thing happened again. This time she kicked me a little higher up the leg.

I fell against the wall, almost weeping with pain and rage. After a few minutes I made up my mind. To hell with her. I had had enough for one day.

Leaving her out, I worked my way along till I had tested all the others. However, I had to pass her on my way back. I stopped and looked at her. I decided to have just one more go. Maybe she did not like my coming from behind. Perhaps if I worked from the side she would not mind so much.

Carefully I squeezed my way between her and the next cow. Once in the space beyond her, I thought, I would be free to do my job. That was my big mistake. As soon as I got there the cow went to work on me. Quickly moving her back end round to cut off my way of escape, she began to kick me from head to foot.

I was desperate. I was trapped. I don't know what made me look up, but there in the thick wall was a hole about two feet square, where the stone had fallen out. I pulled myself up and crawled through, head first. When I got there I found I was looking through into a hay barn. I flung myself through, and landed safely on my back.

Lying there in the hay, bruised and out of breath, I gave up the idea altogether that working for the Ministry was a soft touch.

I was getting slowly to my feet when Mr Bell came in.

'Sorry I had to go out,' he said. He looked at me with interest. I dusted myself down and picked out a few strands of hay from my hair. I told him that I had managed to get the job done.

'Were you having a bit of a kip in here, then?' he asked.

'No, not exactly. I had some trouble with one of your cows.' I told him the story.

Mr Bell listened. His smile got bigger and bigger. By the time I had finished he was doubled up, nearly crying with laughter. This lasted some time, then he took off his cap and wiped his eyes with the lining.

'I can just imagine it,' he said. 'She's a right bitch that one. Bought her cheap at market last spring. It took us a fortnight to get her tied up.' He looked at the hole in the wall. 'And you crawled through. . . .' He went into another fit of laughter. 'Oh dear, oh dear,' he said weakly, 'I wish I had been here!'

19 Eyes closed

My last call was just out of Darrowby. I could hear the church clock striking a quarter past seven as I got out of the car. I was stiff all over. After my 'easy' day working for the Government I felt broken in mind and body. I nearly screamed when I saw another long line of cows' back-sides waiting for me. It was almost dark in the gloom of the cow-shed.

Right, no messing about. I was going to make a quick job of this and get home. So, left hand holding the tail, right hand on the udder, a quick feel around, then on to the next one. Eyes half closed I moved from cow to cow, like a robot.

And at last here it was, the very last one. Left hand on the tail, right hand on the udder. . . . At first my tired brain did not take in the fact that there was something odd here, but there *was* something very odd. A lot of space, something hanging down in two halves instead of four quarters, and no teats to be found!

I woke up suddenly and looked at the animal's side. A huge woolly head turned towards me and two wide-set eyes were looking at me. In the dull light I could just see the ring in the nose.

The farmer, who had been watching me, spoke up, 'You're wasting your time there, young man. There's nothing wrong with *his* bag.'

20 Miss Stubbs

There was a card over the old lady's bed. It said 'GOD IS NEAR'. From where she lay Miss Stubbs could look up and read it.

There was not much more Miss Stubbs could see. Mainly it was just the little room, full of bits and pieces, that had been her world for many years.

The room was on the ground floor, in the front of the cottage. As I came through the wilderness that had once been the garden I could see the dogs watching me. They had jumped up on the old lady's bed. I had been visiting for over a year now and each time I came it was always the same. First, loud barking. Then Mrs Broadwith, who looked after Miss Stubbs, would put all the animals except the one I had come to see into the back kitchen. Then she would open the door to me, and I would go in. Miss Stubbs was in the corner in her bed with the card hanging over it.

She had been there for a long time and would never get up again, but she never spoke to me about her illness and pain. All she worried about was her two cats and three dogs.

Today it was old Prince. I was worried about him too. It was his heart. He was waiting for me and wagging his tail as I came in, pleased as ever to see me.

'I thought I'd give you a ring, Mr Herriot,' Mrs Broadwith said. 'He's been coughing real bad this week. This morning he seemed to be staggering a bit. Still eats well, though.'

'I'll bet he does,' I said. I ran my hands over the rolls of fat on the dog's ribs. 'It would take something really drastic to put old Prince off his food.'

Miss Stubbs laughed from her bed. I sounded his heart, knowing what I was going to hear. They say the heart should go 'Lub-dub, lub-dub', but Prince's went 'Swish-swoosh, swish-swoosh'. There seemed to be nearly as much blood leaking back as was being pumped into the blood stream from his worn-out old heart.

Like all old dogs with heart trouble, Prince always had bronchitis. I listened sadly to all the squeaks and rattles from Prince's chest and I could tell what state his lungs were in. The old dog stood very straight and proud, his tail wagging. He always took it as a great

53

compliment when I checked him over. He was enjoying himself now.

I gave him an injection to help his heart and another to help him rest. 'That will help his heart and breathing, Miss Stubbs,' I said. 'You'll find he'll be a bit dopey for the rest of the day. Carry on with the tablets. I'm going to leave you some more stuff for his bronchitis.'

The next stage of the visit began. Mrs Broadwith brought in a cup of tea and the other animals were let out of the kitchen. There was Ben, a sealyham, and Sally, a spaniel. They were followed by the cats, Arthur and Susie.

It was the usual setting for the many cups of tea I had drunk with Miss Stubbs under the card that hung above her bed.

'How are you today?' I asked her.

'Oh, much better,' she replied straight away, and changed the subject.

She liked to talk about her pets. She spoke a lot, too, about the days when her family was alive.

The things I had heard in the village came back to me. About the rich family who lived in the big house many years ago. Then the business that went wrong, and the sudden loss of money. 'When her father died almost all his money had gone,' one old man had said to me. 'There's not much to live on now.'

Just enough to keep Miss Stubbs and her animals alive and to pay Mrs Broadwith. Not enough to keep the garden dug or the house painted.

21 A sad day

I sat there drinking tea, with the dogs in a row by the
bed-side and the cats on the bed. As I always did, I
felt a bit afraid at the thought of how much depended
on me. The one thing that brought some light into
this brave old woman's life was her pets. This shaggy
bunch loved her so much that their eyes were always
on her face. The snag was they were all so old. I had
them to look after and none of them was less than ten
years old.

They were all of them perky enough, but all of them
showed some signs of old age. Prince had his bad
heart. Sally was beginning to drink a lot and this
made me wonder whether she was starting to have
womb trouble. Ben was getting thinner and thinner
with his kidney trouble.

The cats were better, although Susie was a bit
scraggy. Arthur was the best of the bunch. The only
thing wrong with him was that his teeth got a lot of
scale on them.

My next visit was less than a month later. Mrs
Broadwith had sent for me at six o'clock in the evening.
Ben had collapsed. I jumped straight into my car and
was at the house in less than ten minutes. The barking
broke out as I knocked but I could not hear Ben. As I
went into the little room I saw the old dog lying on his
side, very still, beside the bed.

D O A is what we write in the book. Dead on arrival.
I said, 'Well, it was quick, Miss Stubbs. I'm sure the
old chap did not suffer at all.'

The old lady did not cry. Her face was very sad,

though, when she looked down at her friend of so many years. My idea was to get him out of the house as quickly as I could. I lifted him up. As I was moving away Miss Stubbs said, 'Wait a minute.' She turned on her side and looked at Ben. She reached out and touched his head softly. Then she lay back as I hurried from the room.

I went back and sat by the bed. Miss Stubbs looked out of the window for a few minutes and then said to me, 'You know, Mr Herriot, it will be my turn next.'

'Nonsense!' I said. 'You're just feeling a bit low, that's all. We all do when something like this happens.' I was worried. I had never heard her hint at such a thing before.

'I'm not afraid,' she said. 'I know there's something better waiting for me.' She lay calmly looking at the card on the wall. 'I have only one fear,' she said and her face changed. Fear showed in her eyes and she took my hand. 'It's my dogs and cats, Mr Herriot. I'm afraid I might never see them again when I'm gone and it worries me so. You see, I know I'll see my family again, but . . . but . . .'

'Well, why not your animals?' I asked.

'That's just it,' she said, and for the first time I saw tears on her cheeks. 'Some people say that animals can't go to heaven because they have no souls.'

'I don't believe it,' I said and I patted her hand. 'If having a soul means being able to feel love, then animals are better off than a lot of humans. You've nothing to worry about there.'

'I hope you're right. I lie awake at night thinking about it.'

'I know I'm right, Miss Stubbs. Don't argue with me. They teach vets all about animals' souls,' I said with a smile.

She laughed and said, 'I'm sorry to bore you with this. I won't talk about it again. But before you go I

56

want you to be honest with me. I know you are very young but please tell me. What do you believe? Will my animals go with me?' She stared at me.

I shifted my chair and said, 'Miss Stubbs, I'm afraid I'm a bit foggy about this. But I am sure about one thing: wherever you are going, your animals are sure to go, too.'

She still stared at me but her face was calm. She said, 'Thank you, Mr Herriot. I know you are being honest with me. That is what you really believe, isn't it?'

'I do believe it,' I said. 'With all my heart I believe it.'

22   A new home for old friends

It must have been about a month later that I heard of Miss Stubbs's death. I was on my rounds. A farmer told me that her cottage was up for sale.

'But what about Miss Stubbs?' I asked.

'Went off sudden about three weeks ago,' he said.

'Do you know what's happened to the dogs and cats?' I asked.

'What dogs and cats?'

I cut my visit short. I did not go home, though it was nearly lunch time. Instead I got in my car and drove to the village where Miss Stubbs had lived. I asked the first person I saw where Mrs Broadwith was living. When I knocked on her door she opened it herself.

'Come in, Mr Herriot. It's good of you to call,' she said, and I went inside. 'It was sad about the old lady,' she said. 'She just went in her sleep at the end.'

'What about the animals?' I asked.

'Oh, they're in the garden,' she said calmly. She got up and opened the door. I was so pleased as I watched all my old friends come in.

Arthur was on my knee in a flash, purring away. Prince wagged his tail in delight to see me.

'They look great, Mrs Broadwith. How long are they going to be here?' I asked.

'They're here for good. I think just as much of them as the old lady did. I couldn't be parted from them. They'll have a good home with me as long as they live.'

'This is wonderful,' I said. 'But won't you find them a bit dear to keep?'

'No, you don't have to worry about that. I have some money put away,' she said.

'Well, fine, fine. I'll be looking in now and then to see how they are.' I got up and started for the door.

Mrs Broadwith said, 'There's just one thing. Would you mind popping in to the cottage to collect what's left of your medicines? They're in the front room.'

I took the key and drove along to Miss Stubbs's house. How lifeless the house looked without the dogs' faces at the window.

Nothing had been moved. The bed was still in the same corner. I moved around, picking up half empty bottles, a jar of ointment, the box with old Ben's tablets in – a lot of good they had done him.

When I had got everything I looked round the little room. I would not be coming here any more. At the door I stopped and read for the last time the card that hung over the empty bed.

23   Taking the bull by the horns

I was spending Tuesday evening as I spent all the Tuesday evenings – gazing at the back of Helen Alderson's head. I had joined the Darrowby Music Society. It was a slow way of getting to know her, but I could not think of a better idea.

Since the morning on the high moor when I had set the calf's leg, I had hoped to make another visit to the farm. But the Aldersons seemed to have very healthy animals, sad to say. I had to be content with the thought that there was the visit at the end of the month to take off the plaster. The really crushing blow came when Helen's father rang up. He said that as the calf was getting on so well he had taken off the plaster himself.

That was why I had joined the Music Society. I had seen her going into the meeting one Tuesday night, and had followed her in.

That was weeks ago. I had made no progress at all. I could not remember how many singers had come and gone. At one meeting the local brass band had packed themselves into the little room and they had almost broken my eardrums. However, I had still made no progress with her.

Tonight a string quartet was scraping away. I hardly heard them. My eyes were on Helen. She sat a few rows in front of me, between the two old ladies she always seemed to bring with her. That was part of the trouble. Those two old girls were always with her, cutting out any chance of me talking to Helen alone, even in the half-time break for tea. Nearly everyone at the meetings was elderly, and over everything hung the school-room smell of ink and books and chalk and pencils. It was not the sort of place where you could say, 'Are you doing anything next Saturday?'

The scraping stopped and everybody clapped. Time for tea. I went to the back of the hall with the others, put my threepence on the plate and took my cup of tea and a biscuit. This was when I tried to get near Helen. It was not always easy, because often people would try to stop me and have a talk. Tonight I managed to get myself into the group of people she was in.

She looked at me over her cup of tea and said, 'Good evening, Mr Herriot. Are you enjoying the music?'

Oh, Lord, she always said that – and *Mr Herriot!* What could I do? I did not dare say, 'Call me Jim.' I said, as always, 'Good evening, Miss Alderson. Yes, very nice, isn't it?' Things were really going with a bang.

I ate my biscuit while the old ladies talked about music. It was going to be the same as all the other Tuesdays. I felt beaten.

Then the vicar came over to us and said, 'I'm afraid I have to ask somebody to wash up the cups. Perhaps our two young friends would do it tonight?'

I had never been very fond of washing up, but suddenly it seemed just the thing I wanted to do most. I said, 'Yes, delighted – that is, if it's all right with Miss Alderson.'

Helen smiled and said, 'Of course it's all right. We all have to take a turn, don't we?'

I pushed the trolley of cups and saucers into the scullery. It was a small, cramped room with a sink and a few shelves. There was just about room for the two of us to get inside.

'Would you like to wash or dry?' Helen said.

'I'll wash,' I said and began to run the hot water into the sink. It should not be hard now, I thought, to work my way round to asking her out. I would never have a better chance than this, jammed into this little room together.

But it was surprising how the time went by. Five whole minutes and we had not talked about anything but music, and I had washed up nearly all the cups! The feeling changed to panic when I took the last cup from the soapy water.

It had to be now. I held out the cup to Helen and she tried to take it from me. I held on to it tight while I tried to think what to say. She pulled at it but I held on tight. It was getting like a tug of war. Then I heard a gruff voice that did not sound like mine at all say, 'Can I see you some time?'

For a moment she did not say anything. Was she surprised? Angry? Shocked? She went pink and said, 'If you like.'

I heard that funny voice again, 'Saturday evening?' She nodded, dried the cup and was gone.

I went back to my seat, my heart thudding. I had done it at last, but did she really want to come out? Had I pushed her into it? Still, it was a step forward.

24 John Skipton

Autumn had come. It was going to be another fine day, but there was a chill in the air, to remind us that the hard months lay just ahead. As I sat at breakfast I looked out at the mist, melting away in the early sunshine.

Siegfried was deep in the local paper. 'It says here,'

he said, 'that farmers have no feelings for their animals.'

'They're cruel, you mean?' I said.

'No, not quite, but this chap says that farmers think of their animals only as a means of making money. They don't love them,' Siegfried said.

'It wouldn't do if they were all like Kit Bolton, would it? They'd all go mad,' I said.

Kit was a lorry driver. Like many of the working men of Darrowby, to help feed the family he kept a pig at the bottom of his garden. The trouble was that when killing time came Kit cried for three days. I went into his house at one of these times. His wife and daughter were hard at it cutting up the pig for pies and brawn. Kit sat by the kitchen fire, his eyes full of tears. He took my hand and said, 'I can't bear it, Mr Herriot. He was like a Christian, that pig, just like a Christian.' I shall never forget it.

Siegfried agreed with me when I reminded him of Kit, but he pointed out that Kit was not a full-time farmer. He went on, 'The question is about people who own a large number of animals. Can a dairy farmer milking fifty cows a day get really fond of any of them or are they just a way to make money?'

I thought about it and decided it *was* a matter of numbers. Some of the farmers up in the high farms had only a few cows. They always had names for each of them. They probably did grow fond of their animals, but I did not see how the men with a great many animals could.

Siegfried got up from the table and said, 'I expect you're right. Anyway I'm sending you to see a really big man this morning. John Skipton of Dennaby Close. He's got two horses a bit out of condition. They need their teeth rasping.'

I staggered to the car with a box full of tooth instruments.

Dennaby Close was a very fine house indeed. John Skipton had started as a farm labourer without any education and was now a rich land owner.

It had not happened easily. Old John had a life-time of very hard work behind him, that would have killed most men. A life-time with no room for a wife or family or comfort, but there was more to it than that. He was a marvellous business man. 'When all the world goes one way, I go the other' was one of his sayings. It is true that the Skipton farms had made money in the hard times when others were going broke.

He had won, but some people thought that he had been beaten himself. He had fought against the odds for so many years and driven himself so hard that he just could not stop working. Now that he could enjoy life he just had not got the time. They said that the poorest of his workers lived better than he did.

25 The love of animals

Dennaby Close was a beautiful house. There should have been a beautiful woman in it, but there was only old John. He stumped towards me, his shabby old coat tied round his middle with a bit of string. There were no socks under his heavy boots.

'We'll have to walk down to the river. The horses are down there,' he said to me, and trotted off.

I took the box of instruments from the car. It was a funny thing, but whenever I had heavy stuff to lug about, my patients were always a long way away. This box seemed to be filled with lead.

The old man took a pitch-fork, stabbed a bale of

hay and put it over his shoulder. He set off again at a fast walk. We made our way across the fields. John did not slow down, and I stumbled after him. I puffed and tried not to remember that he was more than fifty years older than I.

I was glad when we got to the flat land at the bottom. My arms felt several inches longer, and I was sweating. Old John looked as cool as when we started. He tossed the hay on to the grass.

The two horses, one a mare, the other a gelding, turned to us at the noise. They were standing in shallow water at the edge of the river. Nose to tail, they were rubbing their chins along each other's backs.

'They're in a nice spot, Mr Skipton,' I said.

'Yes, they keep cool in the hot weather and they've got the barn when the winter comes. They can come and go as they please,' he said.

The sound of his voice brought the horses from the river at a quick trot. As they came near I saw that they were really old. Their coats were flecked with grey. On their faces were many white hairs, and their eyes were sunken.

For all that, they danced around John, stamping their feet. They threw their heads in the air, and pushed his cap over his eyes.

'Get off!' he shouted. 'Daft old beggars.' But I saw that he patted them both fondly.

'When did they last do any work?' I asked.

'Oh, about twelve years ago,' he said.

I stared at him. 'Twelve years! Have they been down here all that time?'

'Yes, just larking about down here, retired like. They've earned it,' he said. For a few moments he stood silent, then he said softly, 'They were two slaves when I was a slave.' He looked at me and in his eyes I read something of the hard times he had shared with the two animals.

I asked him how old they were. He smiled and said, 'You're the vet; you tell me.'

I looked at the mare's teeth.

'Good God!' I gasped, 'I've never seen anything like this.' All the usual ways of judging a horse's age by the state of its teeth buzzed around in my head, but I had never seen teeth as old as this. I laughed, and said, 'It's no good. You'll have to tell me.'

'Well, she's about thirty, and the gelding is a year or two younger. She's had fifteen foals, and never been ill once, except for a bit of tooth trouble. We've had them rasped once or twice, and it's time for them to be done again. They both have a job chewing their food.'

I put my hand into the mare's mouth, grasped her tongue and pulled it out to one side. I felt her back teeth with my hand. The outside edges of the upper teeth were jagged. They were making the inside of her cheeks sore. The lower teeth were making her tongue sore in the same way.

'I'll soon make her more comfortable, Mr Skipton,' I said. 'With these sharp edges rubbed off she'll be as good as new.' I got the rasp out of my heavy box. I held the tongue in one hand and worked at the rough edges of the teeth until they were smoother.

'That's about right,' I said after a few minutes. 'I don't want to make them too smooth or she won't be able to grind her food.' Then I began the same job on the other horse.

When I had finished I put the tools away, and we started on our way back. John was able to go twice as fast now he was not carrying the bale of straw. I panted along behind him, changing the box from hand to hand every few minutes.

About half-way up, the box slipped from my hand, and it gave me a chance to stop for a breather. I looked back and could just see the two horses. They had gone back into the water and were playing together. It all made a lovely picture.

Back in the farm-yard, John stopped. He nodded once or twice and said, 'Thank you, young man,' then turned and quickly walked away.

I was putting the heavy box back in the boot when I got talking to one of the farm-workers. He was sitting in a sunny corner of the farm-yard eating his dinner.

'You've been down to see the two old horses, then? By God, old John should know the way there,' he said. He went on to tell me that John never missed a day in his visits to the two old horses. He always took them something, a bag of corn or some straw for their bedding. For twelve solid years he had kept the horses, and they had not done a stroke of work all that time.

'Yes, he could have got good money if he had sold them as horse flesh,' he said. 'Strange, isn't it?'

'You're right,' I said, 'it is strange.'

On my way home I was thinking just how strange it was. I thought of my talk with Siegfried that morning. We had just about decided that a man with a lot of animals could not be fond of them all, or even a few of them. But John Skipton must have had dozens of animals.

What made him go down that hill-side every day in all weathers? Why had he given them the comfortable life that he had not let himself have?

It could only be love.

26   Out cold

The Dales farmers were all good stock-men. They really knew how to handle animals. This was a great comfort to a vet who does not want to be hurt by animals or slowed down when he works with them.

So this morning I was glad to see the two men holding the cow. It was not a hard job, only an injection. Still, it was good to have two such strong chaps to help me. Maurice Bennison, not tall but as tough as one of his hill beasts, held a horn in his right hand. The fingers of his left gripped the animal's nose. I felt the cow would not jump very far when I pushed the needle in. His brother George had the job of raising the vein. He held a rope round the animal's neck in huge hands like bunches of carrots. He was six feet four inches tall.

'Right, George,' I said, 'tighten up that rope and lean against the cow to stop her coming round on me.' I bent over the big vein in the cow's neck. It was standing up very nicely. I held the needle, feeling the big man's elbow on me as he looked over my shoulder, and pushed it quickly into the vein.

'Lovely!' I said, as the dark blood shot out on to the straw below. 'Let the rope go, George,' I said, 'and for God's sake, get your weight off me!'

I said this because George was resting his full fourteen stone on me instead of on the cow. As I tried to fix the tube to the needle I felt my knees giving way. I shouted again but he did not move.

There could only be one end to it. I fell flat on my face under George. He had fainted at the sight of the blood!

Mr Bennison, hearing the noise, came into the cow-shed just in time to see me crawling out from under his eldest son.

'Get him out quickly!' I gasped, 'before the cow tramples on him!'

Maurice and his father took an ankle each and pulled. George shot out from under the cow, his head banging on the cobbles. They propped him up against the wall. The poor fellow did not look so good.

Mr Bennison felt he had spent too much time on George, however. He said to me, 'Let's get on with the job.'

This made me think of the way many people react to the sight of blood. It seemed to me that more often than not it was the big men who went down.

Were country people softer about this sort of thing than town folk, in spite of having more to do with natural things? I had asked myself this question ever since Sid Blenkinsop had staggered in to see us one night. He had been upset by something.

'Have you got a drop of whisky, Jim?' he asked. I had helped him into a chair and Siegfried had put a glass into his hand. He had been at a first aid talk given by the doctor, he told us.

'He was talking about blood and veins and things,' he groaned. 'God, it was awful!' The fishmonger had fainted after only ten minutes. Sid himself had only just made the door. It had been a real mess.

I think vets must have more trouble in this way than doctors, because if doctors have any cutting up to do they send people to hospital. Vets just have to get their coats off and start work on the spot. It means that the owners of the animals are pulled in as helpers, and see some nasty sights.

I have a very clear memory of a summer evening when I had to open up a cow. The farmer told me that he had been nailing up loose wood in a hen house in the cow field. He was sure the cow had eaten one of the nails he had been using.

The farm was right on the main street of the village. It was the meeting place for the local lads. As I laid out my instruments on a clean towel a row of grinning faces watched from above the half door of the box. There were quite a lot of cheeky shouts as well.

'How would one of you lads like to help?' I asked, when I was about ready. There was even more shouting for a minute or two. Then the door opened and a huge young man with red hair came into the box.

I told him to roll up his sleeves and scrub his hands in a bucket of warm water while I gave the cow a jab of local anaesthetic. When I gave him some forceps and scissors to hold he danced around and roared with laughter, really playing the fool.

'Maybe you'd like to do the job yourself?' I asked.

'OK, I'll have a go,' he said, and the heads above the door gave him a cheer.

The air was thick with earthy jokes, as I touched the cow's flank with my blade. With a quick move I laid open a ten-inch wound. I stood back for a second to admire the clean cut. At the same time I noticed that the laughter and shouting had stopped. Instead there was a strange quiet broken only by a heavy thud from behind me.

'Forceps, please,' I said. Nothing happened. I looked around. The top half of the door was bare – not a head in sight. There was only the red-headed man lying in the middle of the floor. He was out cold. He must have gone over backwards like a felled tree.

The farmer, a bent little man of about eight stone, had been holding the cow's head. He looked at me with a smile, 'Only you and me left, sir.' He tied the cow to a ring in the wall, washed his hands, and took his place at my side.

During the operation he passed me my instruments and swabbed the blood away. He whistled all the time. The only time he said anything was when I showed him the nail that had caused all the trouble. He raised his eyebrows and said 'Hello, hello,' then started whistling again.

27 The Sidlows

The Sidlow family thought very little of vets. In fact, when you came down to it, just about the only person for miles around who knew anything about animals was Mr Sidlow himself. At least, that is what Mr Sidlow thought. If any farmer's cows or horses fell ill it was Mr Sidlow who stepped forward and took over.

Mind you, Mr Sidlow was a just and kind man. He would nurse the animal for five or six days. During this time he would perhaps push half a pound of lard and raisins down the cow's throat three times a day, or cut a bit of its tail to let the bad out. After that he always in the end called the vet. Not that the vet would do any good, but Mr Sidlow liked to give the animal every chance. When the vet came he always found the animal dying, so whatever he did could not save it. So the Sidlows were even more sure that vets were no good.

We were the third firm of vets Mr Sidlow had tried. He had not been pleased with the others, so now it was our turn. He had been with us now for over a year, but all was not happy between us. Siegfried had made him angry on his very first visit.

Mr Sidlow had a horse that was dying, so he had

been pushing raw onions up its back-side. He could not understand why it was so unsteady on its legs. Siegfried had pointed out that if he pushed a raw onion up Mr Sidlow's back-side Mr Sidlow would be unsteady on *his* legs.

It was a bad start, but there were no other vets left. He was stuck with us.

I had been very lucky. I had been in Darrowby for more than a year and had never had to visit the farm. It was always on Siegfried's duty nights that Mr Sidlow had called us out.

When it did come round to my turn, I did not rush off with any great delight, even though the job sounded easy enough. He had a bullock that was choking on a bit of turnip or potato which was stuck in its throat. This can kill the animal, as it stops it bringing up gases, and so it fills up with gases and gets bloated. The vet either makes a hole in the stomach or carefully pushes the bit of food down into the stomach with a long instrument.

The bullock was in a box off the yard. Several of the family had come in with Mr Sidlow and me. All of them had the same stern, unsmiling look as their father. I examined the animal. Nobody said anything.

I would have liked to break the silence but I could not think of anything cheerful to say. I was worried. I could feel the bit of potato easily enough from the out-side, but there was a lot of swelling all around it. Not only that, but there was a bloody foam dripping from the mouth. There was something strange here.

A thought struck me and I said, 'Have you been trying to push the potato down with something?'

Mr Sidlow said, 'Yes, we've tried a bit.' I asked him what he had used.

'A broom handle and a bit of hose pipe. Same as usual,' he said.

That was enough. It would have been nice to be the

first vet to please this man, but I knew when I was beaten. I said to the farmer,

'I'm afraid you've made a hole in the side of the throat. The walls are very thin. I've seen this happen before. The out-look is pretty black.'

'All right,' said Mr Sidlow. 'What are you going to do about it?'

What was I going to do about it? Perhaps in these days I might have tried to mend the tear, pack the wound with the latest drugs and give a lot of injections. But thirty years ago, as I looked at the poor animal in pain, coughing up blood, I knew I was beaten.

'I'm sorry, Mr Sidlow, I can't do anything about it,' I said. I did not need to be told what they were thinking – another useless vet. I went on, 'Even if I moved the potato, the wound would get infected when the beast tried to eat. There's no hope for him. He's in good shape. If I were you I'd have him killed right away.'

At last Mr Sidlow said, 'That beast is not ready for killing yet.'

'No, but you'd be sending him in before long. I'm sure you won't lose much. I tell you what,' I said, trying to be cheerful, 'if I can come into the house, I'll write you a note now. It will say that this animal is healthy, and OK to be used for butcher's meat. Then we'll get the job over. There's really nothing else for it.'

I turned and walked across the yard to the kitchen. Mr Sidlow and the family followed. I wrote the note quickly. As I folded up the note I suddenly felt sure that Mr Sidlow would not take my advice. He meant to take a day or two to see how things turned out. I had a picture in my mind of the big animal trying to eat and drink as he got hungry and thirsty, and not being able to. I could not leave things as they were. I could not risk this happening. I went over to the phone.

'I'll just give the chap at the slaughter-house a ring,' I told Mr Sidlow. I fixed it so that someone would come and shoot the animal and take it away then and there.

'Much better to get it done now,' I said to them all, and got out of the place as fast as I could.

That was my first visit to the Sidlows, and I hoped it would be my last.

28 Mr Sidlow again

But my luck had run out. From then on, every time they sent for a vet it was my turn to be on duty and something went wrong every time. Try as I might I could not do a thing right on that farm. The Sidlows did not think much of vets. They had met some really poor ones in their time, but I was by far the worst.

It got so bad that if I saw any Sidlows in the town I would dive down an alley to miss them.

However, the Sidlows were far from my mind on the Saturday morning that Siegfried asked me if I would go and be one of the vets on duty at a local race meeting at Brawton. He told me there was nothing much to the job. The usual race-course vet would be there and he would keep his eye on me.

Siegfried had not been gone more than a few minutes when there was a call from the race course. One of the horses had fallen while being unloaded from his box. He had damaged his knee, and would I come right away.

In my short stay in Darrowby I had had very little

to do with horses. Siegfried loved horse work, so he did everything in that line that came along.

I was not too happy when I saw the horse. The knee was a terrible mess with the torn skin hanging down in bloody strips. You could see about six inches of the bone laid bare. The beautiful three-year-old held his leg up, trembling.

I gently felt round the joint. I was glad of one thing – it was a quiet animal. He hardly moved as I tried to piece together the jigsaw of skin. Luckily, none of it was missing.

My heart beating, I got down to the job.

I must have stayed there for nearly an hour, carefully pulling the flaps of skin into place. I must have put in dozens of tiny stitches. It's always interesting to mend a ragged wound. I never mind taking pains with it. When I got up at last, I did so slowly like an old man. The stable lad who had been with me the whole time, smiled at me.

'You've made a good job of that,' he said. 'It looks nearly as good as new. I want to thank you, sir. I'm very fond of this horse.'

'Well, I hope he does all right,' I said. 'I'm just going to cover the knee with a bandage and give him a shot against tetanus, and that's it.'

I was packing my gear away in the car when the stable lad asked me, 'Do you bet on horses?'

I laughed and said no, and that I did not know much about racing.

'Well, never mind. I'll tell you something to back this afternoon. Kemal in the first race. He's one of ours and he's going to win,' he said.

'Well, thanks. I'll have half a crown on him,' I said.

The tough little face showed me he did not think much of that. He said, 'No, no, put a fiver on him.' He walked quickly away.

I don't know what madness took hold of me, but

by the time I got back to Darrowby I had made up my mind to do as he said. The chap had been trying to do me a good turn. Maybe from the look of my shabby clothes he thought I needed the money.

I went into the bank and drew out £5: exactly half of the money I had. I had a quick lunch and changed into my best suit. There would be plenty of time to get to the race-course and get my fiver on Kemal before the first race at 2.30.

The phone rang just as I was going out of the house. It was Mr Sidlow. He had a cow that he wanted looking at right away. What luck! But I shook myself. The Sidlow farm was right near Brawton. It should not take long to look at his cow. I could still make it.

When I got there they were clearly surprised to see me looking so smart. We went into the cow-shed. My heart began to sink as Mr Sidlow told me about the trouble he had had with this cow. It had had the runs for some months. He had tried to put it right with ground eggshells in mash to begin with, then he had tried dandelion tea. All to no effect.

One glance at the animal was enough, I was pretty sure it had quite a common wasting disease. Nobody can be quite sure, of course. I grasped her tail and put the thermometer into her rectum. I did not think she had a fever, but it gave me a few minutes to think.

However, in this case I only got about five seconds. Without warning, the thermometer went from my fingers. Some sudden suction had drawn it inside the cow. I ran my fingers round just inside the rectum. Nothing. I pushed my hand inside. Nothing. With a feeling of panic I rolled up my sleeves and felt about – in vain.

There was nothing else for it, I had to ask for a bucket of hot water, soap and a towel. I had to strip off as if I was about to start a big job. I must have looked a real fool.

You cannot think how pleased I was when at last I felt the thermometer in my fingers. I pulled it out, filthy and dripping, and stared down at it.

Mr Sidlow said in a gruff voice, 'Well, what does it say? Has she got a temperature?'

I managed to say that she had not.

I cannot remember much more of that visit. I got myself cleaned up and dressed. I told Mr Sidlow that I thought the cow had a wasting disease, and that nothing could be done for her if this were so. Anyway, I would take away a sample for testing.

I left the farm feeling even more of a sense of failure than ever. I put my foot down hard all the way to Brawton. I roared into the car park at the race-course and grabbed the arm of the car park keeper. 'Has the first race been run?' I gasped.

'Yes, just this minute,' he said. 'Kemal won it, ten to one.'

I walked slowly away. My £5 at ten to one would have won me £50! Nearly a fortune, stolen from me by fate. It was too much. I could forgive Mr Sidlow, I thought, for giving me a long list of hopeless cases that made me feel not much good at my job. I could forgive him for thinking me the biggest idiot in Yorkshire and telling everybody so. But I would never forgive him for losing me that £50.

29 An old suit

At last I had had the courage to ask Helen out for the evening. The trouble was, where was I going to take her? Of course, I must ask Tristan.

Tristan lay back in his favourite arm-chair and

looked at me through a cloud of cigarette smoke. He thought for a moment and then said:

'The Reniston Hotel is the only place. Of course it is very grand. It's the best hotel in the country outside London. But for Helen it's the only possible place. Look, tonight is your big chance, isn't it? You want to impress the girl, don't you? Well, ring her up and tell her you're taking her to the Reniston. The food is wonderful, and there's a dinner dance every Saturday night. Today is Saturday.'

He sat up suddenly and his eyes grew wide. 'Can't you see it, Jim? Soft lights, sweet music and you, full of good food, floating round the floor holding Helen in your arms. The only problem is that it will cost you a packet. If you are ready to spend about two weeks' wages, though, you can have a really good night.'

I had not heard the last bit. I was thinking of the idea of having Helen in my arms.

Tristan broke in, 'There's one thing. Have you got a dinner jacket? You'll need one.'

'I'm not very well off for evening dress. In fact, when I went to Mrs Pumfrey's party I hired a suit. I would not have time for that now. I still have my first and only dinner suit,' I said, 'but I got it when I was about seventeen. I'm not sure I'll be able to get into it now.'

Tristan said,

'That doesn't matter, Jim. As long as you're wearing the proper gear they'll let you in.'

We went upstairs and I tried the suit on. I had been quite a hit in this suit at the college dances when I was a student. Even then it had been a bit tight. Now it looked very old and very old-fashioned.

My troubles really started when I got the suit on. I had put on weight while I had been in Darrowby. The jacket would not reach across my stomach by about six inches. I seemed to have got taller, too.

There was a big gap between the bottom of my waistcoat and the top of my trousers. The trousers were skin tight over my back-side, but baggy in the legs.

We decided to call Mrs Hall, to ask her what she thought of the suit. She was the sort of woman who hardly ever smiled or showed any feeling. The look on her face never seemed to change, but when she saw me her face began to twitch. After a struggle with herself she managed to be very down to earth about the suit.

'If I let the waist out a bit at the back, Mr Herriot, that will work wonders. I'll put a link button across the front of the jacket, then that will be all right. Mind you, there will still be a bit of a gap, but not enough to worry you. I'll give the whole suit a good press. That makes all the difference in the world,' she said.

30 A night out

I have never been too fussy about the way I look, but that night I really went to work on myself. I scrubbed myself and rubbed in after-shave, and did my hair at least a dozen times before I thought it looked OK. Tristan brought in my suit, still hot from the ironing board.

He helped me get dressed. The high, old-fashioned collar gave the most trouble. He nearly strangled me, trapping the flesh of my neck under the stud.

At last I was ready. Tristan slowly looked me over very carefully. I had never seen him look so serious.

'Fine, Jim, fine – you look great. It's not everybody who can wear a dinner jacket as well as you do. Hang on a minute and I'll get your overcoat.'

I went to pick up Helen at the farm. As I got out of the car out-side her house I felt rather nervous. When I had come here before it had been as a vet. This was not the same thing at all. I had come to take this man's daughter out. He might not like it. He might not like me.

I was shown into the kitchen by Helen's young brother. The boy had a hand over his mouth, trying to hide a wide grin. He seemed to think something was funny. Helen's young sister, sitting at a table doing her home-work, was hiding her smile in a book.

Mr Alderson was sitting by the fire reading a farming paper.

'Come in, young man, and sit by the fire,' he said. Suddenly I thought that he must often have to talk to young men who were calling for his daughter. This thought did not make me feel happier.

I sat down at the other side of the fire and Mr Alderson went back to reading his paper. The clock ticked. I looked at the fire until my eyes ached, then I looked at all the pictures on the walls.

After about a year, or so it seemed, Helen came into the room.

She wore a blue dress, without shoulder straps. The kind that seems to stay up by magic. Her dark hair shone. Over one white arm she held her coat.

I felt faint. She looked marvellous. She gave me a smile and walked towards me saying, 'Hello, I hope I haven't kept you waiting too long.'

I mumbled something and helped her on with her coat. She kissed her father, who did not look up, but waved his hand. I could hear the children giggling. We went out. In the car I felt very tense for the first mile or two, and found myself talking about the weather. I had begun to relax a bit when I drove over a little bridge into a dip in the road. Suddenly the car stopped. There was something else. My feet and ankles were freezing cold.

'My God!' I shouted. 'We've run into a bit of flooded road. The water is right into the car. I'm terribly sorry about this. Your feet must be soaked.'

Helen laughed. 'Yes, I am a bit wet, but it's no good sitting about like this. Hadn't we better start pushing?'

Getting out into the black, icy water was a nightmare, but there was no escape. Between us we managed to push the little car out of the water. I dried the plugs by the light of a torch and got the engine going again.

Helen shivered as we got back into the car. 'I'm afraid I'll have to go home and change my shoes and stockings. So will you,' she said.

Back at the farm Mr Alderson was still deep in his farming paper. When he knew that I had come to borrow a pair of his shoes and socks, he threw down the paper with a grunt. He rose groaning from the chair, and muttered to himself as he went upstairs.

Helen followed him. I was left alone with the two children. They looked at my wet trousers with great delight. I had wrung most of the water out of them, but the fine crease that Mrs Hall had put in them had gone. They looked very strange, hanging down in a wide, wet mass from below the knee. As I stood by the fire to dry them, steam rose around me. The children stared at me with wide eyes; this was a big night for them.

Mr Alderson came back with some shoes and rough socks. I pulled on the socks quickly, but shrank back when I saw the shoes. They were a pair of very old-fashioned dancing slippers, made of shiny leather, with wide black silk bows on top.

Mr Alderson had dug himself deep into his chair

again and found his place in his paper. I did not dare ask for another pair of shoes. I put them on.

We took another road to avoid the floods. I kept my foot down so within half an hour we were well on our way. I began to feel better. We were making good time and the little car was going well. I was just thinking we would not be all that late when the steering wheel began to drag to one side. We had a puncture.

I had become an expert at changing wheels as I had a puncture most days. I was out of the car in a flash. Working like a demon I put on the spare wheel. I tried not to notice that this tyre was in exactly the same state as the other one. When we got to the Reniston I did not take my car to the front entrance, but hid it away at the back of the car park. There were too many Bentleys at the front. We trod without a sound on the thick carpet of the entrance hall.

We parted there to get rid of our coats. In the men's cloakroom I scrubbed hard at my oily hands. It did not do much good.

I looked up in the mirror at the attendant waiting behind me to hand me a towel. He stared down at the wide bows on my shoes and the crumpled trouser bottoms. As he handed me over the towel he smiled. I felt I had brought a little extra colour into his life.

I met Helen in the entrance hall, and we went over to the desk.

'What time does the dinner dance start?' I asked.

The girl looked surprised and said, 'I'm sorry, sir, there's no dance tonight. We only have them once a fortnight.'

I turned to Helen in dismay, but she smiled and said, 'It doesn't matter. I don't really care what we do.'

'We can have dinner, anyway,' I said. I tried to speak cheerfully, but I was beginning to wonder whether anything was going to go right. I felt pretty low, and my first sight of the dining-room did not help.

It looked as big as a football field, and was very grand. At the tables sat a lot of beautiful women and handsome men. They all looked very rich. I saw with horror that there was not another dinner jacket in sight.

The head waiter, who looked as if he had royal blood, came towards us and offered to show us to a table. I had a struggle not to call him 'sir'.

He began to make his royal way between the tables. Helen and I followed him. It was a long way to the table. I tried not to see the heads that turned to have a second look at me as I passed.

When we reached the table a swarm of waiters sprang upon us. They pulled out chairs for us, sat us down, shook out our napkins and put them on our laps. I began to feel really low from then on. The evening had been a disaster and felt as if it was going to get worse. I must have been mad to come to this smart place dressed like something out of a jumble sale. I was hot as hell in the dreadful suit and the stud was biting into my neck.

I tried to hold the menu card so that my dirty nails did not show. I ordered for us and, as we ate, talked to Helen as brightly as I could. But somehow we could not think of much to talk about. It seemed that only Helen and I were quiet among all the laughter and talk.

Worst of all, I kept thinking that Helen had never really wanted to come out with me anyway. She had only come because she did not like to say no. She was getting through a boring date as best she could.

The drive home was pretty quiet, too. By the time we drew up out-side the farm my head had begun to ache.

We shook hands and Helen thanked me for a lovely

evening. Her voice shook and she did not look very happy. I said good night, got into the car and drove away.

31 A Great Dane

There did not seem much point in a millionaire doing the football pools to me. So you can imagine how surprised I was to find out how important they were to Harold Denham. He was devoted to them. He knew nothing about football, however. He had never been to a match and could not name one football player. When he found out that I was keen on football he was very pleased. The fact that I could talk about Preston North End and Everton, and knew about Scottish teams as well, made him treat me with even greater respect than he had done before.

Of course we had first met over his animals. He had dogs, cats, rabbits, budgies and goldfish. This meant I was often called to the dusty big house that belonged to him. Its tall towers peeped above the woods around it and could be seen for miles around Darrowby.

When I first knew him my visits were just run of the mill. Perhaps his terrier had cut its paw, or one of the old cats had a chill. Later on I began to wonder. He called me out so often on a Wednesday and the excuse was often a bit thin. I began to suspect there was nothing wrong with the animal, but Harold was having trouble with his eight draws or the easy six.

I could never be quite sure, but it was funny how he always met me with the same words, 'Ah, Mr Herriot, how are your pools?'

He had said this ever since I had won £1 on the three draws one week. I shall never forget his face when I showed him the little slip from Littlewoods and the postal order. That was the only time I won anything, but it still made me an expert in his eyes. Harold never won anything ever.

The Denham family had been people of note in Yorkshire for years. They were gentlemen farmers who used their money to build up rich money-making farms.

Harold had dropped out at an early age. All day and every day he pottered around his house and untidy land. He was not interested in the world out-side. I don't think he thought about other people very much, which was just as well. Most people thought he was not quite right in the head.

However, he was kind and friendly to me. I enjoyed going to his house. He and his wife ate all their meals in the kitchen. In fact they seemed to spend most of their time there, so I always went round to the back of the house.

This time it was to see his Great Dane bitch who had just had puppies and did not seem well. As it was not Wednesday I felt there really might be something wrong with her. Harold made his usual remark.

'I wonder if you could help me, Mr Herriot,' he said as we left the kitchen and walked along a passage. 'I'm looking for an away winner, and I wondered about Sunderland and Aston Villa?'

'Well, I'm not sure, Mr Denham,' I replied. 'Sunderland are a good side, but I happen to know that Raich Carter's aunt is not too well. It could easily affect his game on Saturday.'

Harold looked sad and nodded his head a few times. Then he looked at me sharply for a few seconds and broke into a shout of laughter.

'Ah, Mr Herriot, you're pulling my leg again,' he

said, and went off along the passage, chuckling.

He led me through the big house into a little gun-room. The Great Dane was lying on a dog-bed raised a little off the ground.

Harold patted the dog's head and said, 'She had her puppies yesterday and she's got a nasty dark discharge. She's eating well, but I'd like you to look her over.'

Great Danes as a breed are usually placid animals and the bitch did not move as I took her temperature. She lay on her side, happily listening to the squeals of her family. The little blind puppies climbed over each other to get at her teats.

'Yes, you're right about the discharge, and she's got a slight fever,' I said. I felt her stomach. 'I don't think there's another puppy there, but I'd better have a feel inside her to make sure. Could you bring me some warm water, some soap and a towel, please?'

As the door shut behind Harold I looked around the gun-room. It was not much bigger than a cupboard. There were no guns as Harold did not agree with shooting. I stood there for about ten minutes, wondering why Harold was taking so long. Then I turned to look at a picture on the wall. I heard a sound behind me.

It was a faint, deep growl. I turned and saw the bitch rising slowly from her bed. All the time she glared at me without blinking. For the first time in my life I knew what people mean by blazing eyes.

She thought I was after her pups, of course. After all, her master had gone and there was only this stranger standing in the corner of the room. One thing was sure – she was going to come at me any second. I was glad that I was standing right by the door. Carefully I moved my hand towards the handle. The bitch rose slowly from her bed. I had almost reached the handle when I made the mistake of making a quick grab for it. Just as I touched the handle the bitch came out of the bed like a rocket and sank her teeth into my wrist.

I hit her over the head with my right fist and she let go and bit me high up on the inside of the left thigh. This really made me yell out. I don't know what would have happened if I had not grabbed hold of the only chair in the room. It was old and not very strong but it saved me.

The rest of my spell in the gun-room was rather like a lion tamer act. If anybody had been there to see it they would have found it very funny. At the time, with that great animal stalking round that tiny room, the blood running down my leg and only an old chair to keep the dog away, I did not feel a bit like laughing.

Every few seconds the bitch would throw herself at me. I would dance about, pushing her away with my chair. Once she forced me back against the wall, chair and all. Standing on her hind legs she was as tall as I. I had a close-up of the wide, growling jaws.

My biggest worry was that the chair was beginning to break up. I tried not to think what would happen if it fell to bits. But I was working my way back to the door. I felt the handle at my back. I turned the handle. I knew I had to do something very quickly. I threw what was left of the chair at the bitch and dived out of the room.

I was sitting on the floor looking at my wounds when I saw Harold coming towards me with a basin of hot water and a towel. I knew now why he had been so long. He had been wandering about like that all the time. He had been lost in his own house. Or perhaps he had been worrying about his four aways.

At home I had to put up with some rude remarks about the way I was walking. Later on in my bedroom, however, the smile left Siegfried's face as he looked at my leg.

'Right up there, by God,' he said. 'You know, James, we've often made jokes about what a savage dog might do to us one day. Well, I'll tell you, boy, it damned near happened to you.'

32 Tristan's plan

As I waited for Siegfried to give me my morning list I pulled my scarf higher until it covered my eyes. I turned up the collar of my coat and put on a pair of woollen gloves. A biting north wind was driving the snow past the window, hiding everything with big swirling flakes.

Siegfried bent over the day book. He began to write on a pad. 'I'd better go and see Scruton's calf,' he said. 'You've been looking after it, I know, but I'm going right past the door. Can you tell me about it?' he said.

'Yes, it's been breathing a bit fast and running a temperature of 103. I don't think there's any pneumonia there. In fact it may be developing diphtheria. It has a bit of swelling on the jaw, and the throat glands are up.'

All the time I was speaking Siegfried went on writing on the pad. He stopped only once to speak softly to Miss Harbottle, our secretary. Then he looked up and said, 'Pneumonia, eh? How have you been treating it?'

'No, I said I didn't think it was pneumonia,' I replied. 'I've been giving it injections. And I left some cream to be rubbed on to its throat.'

But Siegfried was writing again. He said nothing

till he had made two lists. He tore one from the pad and gave it to me.

'Right, you've been rubbing cream on to the animal's chest. I suppose it might do a bit of good,' he said.

'They're rubbing it on the calf's throat, not his chest,' I said. But Siegfried had started to tell Miss Harbottle the order of his visits.

Finally he came away from the desk and said, 'Well, that's fine. Let's get on.' But half-way across the floor he stopped and asked, 'Why the devil are you rubbing cream on the calf's throat?'

'Well, I thought it might bring the swelling down a bit,' I said.

'But, James, why should there be any swelling there? Don't you think the cream would do more good on the chest?' Siegfried said.

'No, I don't. Not in a case of calf diphtheria,' I said.

Siegfried put his head on one side and smiled at me. He put his hand on my shoulder.

'My dear old James, perhaps it would be a good thing if you started at the beginning of the story. Take all the time you want. There's no hurry. Speak slowly and then you won't get in a muddle. You told me you were treating a calf for pneumonia. Now, take it from there.'

I began to get rather angry, but managed not to show it. I took a deep breath and said, 'Look, I told you right at the start that I did not think there was any pneumonia. I suspect early diphtheria. There was a bit of fever – 103.'

Siegfried was looking past me at the window. 'God, just look at that snow,' he said. 'We're going to have some fun getting around today.' He pulled his eyes back to my face and said,

'Don't you think with a temperature of 103 you should give it some injections? I don't like to seem bossy, James. Just an idea, but it does sound to me as if you might try some injections.'

'But, hell, I *am* using injections,' I shouted. 'I told you that to start with, but you weren't listening. I've been trying to get this across to you, but what chance have I got . . .?'

'Come, come, dear boy. Come, come. No need to get upset,' said Siegfried, his face shining with kindness and goodwill. I just managed to stop myself giving him a kick on the shin.

'James, James,' he went on, 'I'm sure you've been trying to tell me about this case, in your own way. But we haven't all got the gift of getting things over to people. You're a very good chap, but you must work harder at this. You must plan ahead what you want to say, and get all your facts straight and in the right order. Then you won't get mixed up, as you've been this morning. You'll get it in time, I'm sure.' He gave me a friendly wave of the hand and was gone.

Quickly I walked into the stock room. Seeing a big, empty box on the floor I gave it a good kick. I put so much anger into it my foot went clean through the cardboard. I was getting my foot out when Tristan came in. He had heard us talking.

As he saw me trying to shake the box loose he asked, 'What's up, Jim? Has my big brother been getting under your skin?'

'I don't know why he should be getting under my skin now,' I said. 'I've known him quite a long time and he's always been the same. It's never upset me before. Not like this, anyway. Any other time I'd laugh that sort of thing off. What the hell is wrong with me?'

Tristan looked at me for a moment and then said, 'There's nothing much wrong with you, Jim. I can tell you one thing. You've been just a bit on edge since you went out with that Helen.'

'Oh, God, don't remind me,' I groaned and shut my eyes. 'Anyway, I've not seen her or heard from her since, so that's the end of that. I can't blame her.'

'Yes, that's all very well,' said Tristan. 'But look at you. All right, you had a bad evening and she's given you up. Well, so what? Do you know how many times I've been given up?'

'Given up? I never even got started,' I said.

'Very well then. Forget it, lad, and get out into the big wide world. You've got to live a little. Think of all the lovely girls in Darrowby. You can hardly move for them,' he said.

He went on: 'Tell you what, why don't you let me fix something up? A nice little foursome, just what you need.'

'Oh, I don't know. I'm not keen really.'

'Nonsense!' Tristan said. 'I don't know why I haven't thought of it before. Living like a monk is bad for you. Leave it all to me.'

I went to bed early that night. About eleven o'clock Tristan came into my room. He smelt strongly of cigarettes and beer.

'I've got some good news for you,' he said. 'You remember Brenda?'

'That nurse I've seen you around with?' I asked.

'The very same. Well, she's got a friend, Connie, who's even more beautiful. The four of us are going dancing on Tuesday night.'

'You mean me too?' I asked.

'You're going to have the best time you've ever had. I'll see to that,' he said, as he blew a last blast of smoke into my face and left, laughing to himself.

33 The Rudd family

I had first met Dick Rudd during the last winter. He stood on the doorstep on the kind of black morning when country vets wonder why they ever took up their jobs.

I shivered in my pyjamas at the open front door as the rain beat down. A small man in a woolly hat and an old army great coat was there, leaning on his bike.

'Sorry to ring your bell at this hour,' he said. 'My name's Rudd, Birch Tree Farm. I've got a cow calving and she's not getting on with the job. Will you come?'

I looked closer at the thin face. The rain trickled down his cheeks and dripped from the end of his nose. I told him I'd be along right away. I offered him a lift in the car, as his farm was about four miles away, but he said no. He would have to come back for his bike in any case.

I helped his cow give birth to a fine calf that first morning. Later, drinking a cup of tea in the kitchen, I met all the young Rudds. There were seven of them, and they were older than I expected. Their ages ranged from 20-odd down to about 10. I had not thought of Dick as middle-aged. He had seemed to be a man in his thirties from his perky manner and the way he moved. But as I looked at him I could see his hair was going grey and he had wrinkles round his eyes.

When they were first married, the Rudds had wanted their children to be boys. They had worried when the first five all turned out to be girls. But they kept trying and had been delighted at last to have two fine boys. A farmer farms for his sons and Dick Rudd had something to work for now.

The girls were all big, tall and good looking. The boys were strong and chunky, and looked as if they were going to be huge. I kept looking from them to their tiny mother and father, and wondering how they had managed to get such children.

Dick always called the vet if he had a problem, even if it was only a small one, so I was often at Birch Tree Farm. After every visit I was asked into the house for a cup of tea. Then the whole family stopped work to watch me drink it. Everything I said was met with nods and smiles all round.

None of the Rudds had an easy life, but it did not seem to matter to them. They were all very happy with their lot. We had grown to think of each other as friends and I was very proud of this.

Whenever I left the farm I found something on the seat of my car, a couple of home-made cakes or a few eggs. I don't know how Mrs Rudd spared them, but she always did.

Dick had one great dream – to own a first-class dairy herd of cows. Without money behind him he knew it would be a slow business, but he had set his heart on it. It might not be in his lifetime, but some time, perhaps when his sons were grown up.

I was there to see the very start of it.

34 Strawberry

Dick stopped me on the road one morning and asked me to go up to his place with him. By the look on his face I knew that something big had happened. He led me into the cow-shed without saying anything. I stared at a really splendid cow.

Dick's herd was rather a poor one. Many of the cows were old animals sold off by better-off farmers because they were not doing so well. Others had been reared by Dick from calves and were rough-haired and scruffy. Yet half-way down the cow-shed, not at all like the rest of the cows, was what seemed to me to be a perfect Dairy Short-horn cow.

'Where did she come from, Dick?' I asked, staring. He told me he had bought her from the biggest pedigree breeders in the Dales. I did not ask him whether he had borrowed the money from the bank or whether he had been saving up for years just for this. They had decided to call her Strawberry.

I knew that I was looking not just at a cow but at the beginning of the new herd. I was looking at Dick Rudd's hopes for the future.

It was about a month later that he phoned me. 'I want you to come and look at Strawberry for me,' he said. 'She's been grand, tipping the milk out, but there's something wrong with her this morning.'

The cow did not look ill. In fact she was eating when I looked her over. But I noticed she found it a bit hard to swallow. Her temperature was normal and her lungs were clear. But when I stood by her head I could just hear a faint snoring sound.

'It's her throat, Dick. There's a chance she's got an abscess coming in her throat.' I spoke lightly, but I was not happy. Abscesses in the throat were nasty things. It was always hard to get to them, and they make it hard for the animal to breathe. I had been lucky with the few I had seen. They had either been small and gone away or they had burst themselves.

I gave Strawberry a shot of Prontosil and said to Dick, 'I want you to bathe here, just behind the ear, with hot water. Rub this ointment well in afterwards. You may help to burst the abscess that way. Do this at least three times a day.'

I kept looking in on her over the next ten days. I could tell the abscess was growing. The cow was not really ill, but she was eating a lot less. She was thinner and she was giving less milk. I felt helpless. I knew it was only a matter of waiting for the abscess to burst but it was taking a long time to do it.

It happened that just then Siegfried had to be away for a week and for a few days I was working at full stretch. I hardly had time to think of Dick's cow. He biked to see me one morning. He was cheerful as usual but I could tell he was worried.

'Will you come and see Strawberry? She's gone right downhill over the last three days. I don't like the look of her,' he said.

I drove quickly over to his place, and I got there before he was over half-way home. I stopped dead when I saw Strawberry. I stared at what had once been a show cow. She was as thin as a rake. I could hear her breathing all over the cow-shed. Her scared eyes were fixed on the wall in front of her. Now and then she gave a little cough which made her dribble.

I must have stood there a long time because Dick came into the cow-shed and stood next to me.

'Hell, Dick, I'm sorry. I had no idea she had got to this state. I can't believe it,' I said. He told me it had happened suddenly. He had never known a cow change so quickly. I told him that the abscess must be right at its peak, and that it was almost blocking Strawberry's throat now. That was why she found it so hard to breathe.

As I spoke the cow began to tremble and I thought she would fall, but she did not. I looked at Dick and said, 'I think it's just got to burst tonight.'

'And if it doesn't, she'll die tomorrow,' he said. I must have looked very sad because he suddenly grinned and said, 'Never mind, lad, you've done everything anybody could do.'

But as I walked away I was not so sure. Mrs Rudd met me at the car. It was her baking day and she pushed a little loaf into my hand. It made me feel worse.

35   A shot in the dark

That night I sat alone and thought. Siegfried was still away. I had nobody to turn to. I wondered what I was going to do with that cow of Dick's in the morning. By the time I went to bed I had decided that if the abscess had not burst I would have to go in behind her jaw bone with the knife.

I knew just where the abscess was, but it was a long way in. I tried not to think of the main artery and the jugular vein, but I kept dreaming about them. I was awake by six o'clock, and got up. Without washing or shaving I drove out to the farm.

As I crept into the cow-shed I saw with dismay that Strawberry's stall was empty. So that was that. She was dead. I was turning away when Dick came in.

'I've got her in a box the other side of the yard. I thought she might be a bit more comfortable there,' he said.

I almost ran across the yard. As we came up to the door of the box we heard the sound of the dreadful breathing. Strawberry was off her legs now. She lay on her chest, her head right out in front of her, her nostrils wide open, fighting for breath.

But she was alive.

'Dick,' I said, 'I've just got to get at that abscess. It isn't going to burst in time, so it's now or never. But there's one thing I want you to know. The only way I can think of doing it is by going in from behind the jaw. I've never done this before. I've never seen it done before and I've never heard of anybody doing it. If I cut one of those veins in there it will kill her in a minute.'

'She can't last much longer anyhow,' said Dick. 'There's nothing to lose. Get on with it.'

There was no need to tie Strawberry down as you usually have to with big animals. She was too far gone. I just pushed her gently and she rolled over on her side and lay still.

Quickly I gave her a shot to freeze the area from under the ear to behind the jaw. Then I laid out the instruments.

'Stretch her head right out and slightly back, Dick,' I said. I got down in the straw. I cut the skin, cut through the muscle and held the wound open. I worked out in my mind the exact spot to hit. But as I held the sharp knife over the small place my hand began to shake. I tried to steady it, but I could not. In fact, I was too scared to cut any more. I put the knife down and picked up a long pair of forceps. I pushed them down through the hole I had made. It seemed I had gone a long way when I saw a thin trickle of pus coming out. I could hardly believe it. I was in the abscess.

Carefully I opened the forceps as wide as I could to make the hole bigger, so that it could drain. As I did so the trickle became a stream which gushed over my hand. It ran down the cow's neck and on to the straw. I stayed quite still until it had stopped. Then I took out the forceps.

Dick said, 'Now what?'

'Well, I've emptied the thing, Dick,' I said. 'She should soon be a lot better. Let's roll her on to her chest again.'

When we had got the cow settled comfortably again, I had a good look at her. Surely she must be getting better? But Strawberry looked just the same, and her breathing had not changed.

I began to wash the dirty instruments in a bucket of hot water. 'I know what it is. We've got to wait for the walls of the abscess to go down. They're thick and hard because it's been there so long.'

But I was still worried.

Next day I made my way across the yard, wondering what would greet me. I threw open the door wide.

Strawberry was standing there, eating hay from the rack. Not just eating, but jerking it through the bars as cows do when they are really enjoying their food. It looked as if she could not get it down fast enough. I went into the box, shut the door behind me and sat down in the straw in the corner. I had waited a long time for this. I was going to enjoy it.

The cow was still a walking bag of bones, of course. As she stood she trembled with weakness. But there was a light in her eye, and the way she ate made me sure that she would fight her way back to her old self.

I do not know how long I sat there, but I enjoyed

every minute. It took me some time to take in that what I was watching was really happening.

That cow was amazing. I saw her three weeks later and her bones were covered in flesh again, her skin shone and, most important, she was giving lots of milk again.

I was very pleased, I can tell you.

36 Money

There is one side of a vet's life that isn't talked about in the books he has to swot up. It has to do with money. Most farmers are no trouble at all when it comes to paying their bills, but not all. About one in every ten of them tries to get out of paying altogether.

We had our share of bad payers in Darrowby. They were only a small problem but they were always there. Siegfried did not seem to worry too much, except when the three-monthly bills went out. Then it really got through to him. Sometimes he thought up some very strange ideas to try to solve some of the problems of poor payers. Like the method he thought up for Dennis Pratt.

Dennis was a fat little man who thought very highly of himself. He owed us quite a lot of money. We had managed to get five pounds out of him, but this was more than a year ago. Since then nothing more had happened. Siegfried did not know what to do, as Dennis was such a nice, cheerful man. He was always laughing, or about to laugh.

After a job he always asked us in to try some of Mrs Pratt's baking. In fact, on cold days he used to keep a flask of hot coffee ready for us, if we were expected. He had a very good habit of pouring rum into the cup before pouring in the coffee.

'You can't put a man like that in court,' Siegfried said. 'But we've got to find some way of getting some money out of him.' He thought for a few moments and then said in an excited voice:

'I think I've got it, James! You know it's quite possible that Dennis just never thinks of paying a bill. I'm going to make him think about it. The bills have just gone out and I'm going to offer to meet him here on market day, at two o'clock. I'll say I want to talk to him about his cows. He'll be right in the middle of all the farmers paying their bills, and I'll leave him with them for half an hour or so. I'm sure it will put the idea into his head.'

I felt a bit doubtful. I had known Siegfried long enough to know that some of his ideas were very good and some were useless.

My doubts must have shown on my face, because Siegfried laughed and said, 'Don't look so worried. We can only try. It'll work. Just you wait and see.'

On market day I was looking out of the window when I saw Dennis coming our way. I let him in at the front door.

Siegfried sat him next to Miss Harbottle's desk. Then he left him saying he had to go to see a dog that was in the surgery. I stayed behind to answer any questions and to see what would happen. I had not long to wait. The farmers came in, a steady stream of them, holding their cheque books.

It was the usual sort of bill-paying day, with the usual share of moans. One man asked for something to be taken off his bill, but Miss Harbottle fixed him with a cold eye and said, 'This bill has been owing for a year. You should be paying us interest. I only take something off when a bill is paid quickly. It's too bad of you to let it run on for all this time.'

Dennis, sitting listening, agreed with every word. He shook his head at the farmer and turned to me with a very shocked look on his face.

One old man said, 'I'm sorry I've missed paying for a few months. The vets always come out right away when I call for them, so I reckon it's not fair to keep them waiting for their money.'

I could see that Dennis thought this was very true. He nodded several times and gave the old man a big smile.

Dennis was right in the thick of it. He watched as the farmers wrote out their cheques. He looked with interest at the neat bundles of notes being put away in the desk drawer. I kept making little remarks like, 'It's nice to see the money coming in. We can't carry on without that, can we?'

When the crowd began to thin out a bit Siegfried came in and I left to do my rounds.

When I got back Siegfried was eating his supper. He did not say anything about Dennis and soon I could wait no longer.

'Well, what about Dennis? How did it go?' I asked.

'Oh, fine. We had a good talk about his cows. I'm going out there on Tuesday morning to try a new treatment on his herd,' Siegfried said. I asked if he had shown any signs of paying his bill.

'No, never a sign.' He put his knife down and with a sad look said, 'It didn't work, did it?'

'Oh well, never mind. As you said, we can only try,' I said. Then I went on, 'There's something else, Siegfried. I'm afraid you're going to be angry about this. I know you've told me never to give stuff to people who don't pay, but he talked me into letting him have a few bottles of fever drink. I don't know what came over me.'

'He did, did he?' Siegfried stared into space for a moment and then gave a sad smile. 'Well, you can forget about that. He got six tins of stomach powder out of me.'

37 An evening with Tristan

Tristan was used to waiting out-side the hospital for the nurses to come off duty. He was to be found there on several nights of the week. On the other hand, this was the first time I had been with him.

At half past seven he gave me a nudge. Two girls had come out of the hospital and down the steps. Tristan said, 'Come on, Jim, here they are. That's Connie on the left. Lovely girl.'

We went over and Tristan told them who I was, with his usual charm. I had to admit that I was start-ing to feel better already. There was something very cheering in the way the two girls looked up at me with parted lips and shining eyes.

They were alike, except for their hair. Brenda was very dark, but Connie was fair, with gold and red lights in her hair. Both of them seemed bursting with health – fresh cheeks, white teeth and lively eyes.

Tristan opened the back door of the car and said, 'Be careful in there with him, Connie. He looks quiet, but he's a devil with women. He's known far and wide as a great lover.'

The girls giggled and looked at me with even more interest. Tristan got in and we set off at break-neck speed.

As we drove off through the dark countryside I listened to Tristan, who was in top form. Perhaps he was trying to cheer me up, or perhaps he just felt that way. The girls laughed with delight at everything he said. I could feel Connie shaking against me. She was sitting very close, with a long stretch of seat the other side of her. The little car swung round a sharp corner. It threw her against me. She stayed there with her head on my shoulder. I felt her hair against my cheek.

I put my arm around Connie and she lifted her face to me. I kissed her. Tristan was singing in the front seat. Brenda was giggling. The old car rattled over the rough road.

We came at last to Poulton, a village on the way to nowhere. This was where the dance was to be held, but Tristan had other plans first.

'There's a lovely little pub here,' he said. 'We'll just have a jar to get us in the mood.' In we went.

It was just a large square whitewashed room, with a black cooking-range. A bright fire burnt in the range and a long high-backed settle faced it.

We hurried over to the settle. We had the place to ourselves. The landlord came in. His cheerful face lit up at the sight of Tristan and he said:

'Now then, Mr Farnon, are you well?'

Tristan told him that he was never better, and then turned to me and said, 'Mr Peacock here keeps some of the finest draught beers in Yorkshire. I'd like you to tell me what you think of it, Jim. Perhaps you would be kind enough as to bring us two pints and two halves, Mr Peacock.'

There was no question of asking the girls what they would like to drink, but they seemed quite happy. The landlord came puffing back from the cellar, carrying a tall white jug. He poured us each a glass of beer, with a white head on each glass.

Tristan took his first sip and then shut his eyes. A beautiful smile spread across his face. Then he said: 'Keeping beer in the wood is a skilful business, but you, Mr Peacock, are an artist.'

The landlord lowered his eyes at such praise.

Tristan and the girls soon finished their beers. With an effort I got my own pint down and the white jug went round our glasses again.

Time passed and the landlord kept revisiting the cellar with his jug. In fact, a long time later, as I drank my eighth pint, I thought Tristan had been right – I had been needing this.

It suddenly struck me that Connie was one of the most beautiful girls I had ever seen. Back there in the street out-side the hospital she had seemed pretty but I had failed to see how perfect her skin was. I had missed seeing the grand depths of her eyes and her wonderful hair, catching lights of gold and bronze from the fire. I had missed the laughing mouth, shining even teeth and little pink tongue. She hardly ever stopped laughing, except to drink her beer. Everything I said was witty, and she looked at me all the time as if she thought I were the most marvellous man in the world. It did me a great deal of good.

As the beer flowed, time slowed down. There was no past and no future, only Connie and the warm, trouble-free present.

I was quite surprised when Tristan called for one for the road. Then we shook hands with Mr Peacock as if he were our greatest friend in the world, and left for the dance.

38 The dance

After the lights in the pub the darkness out-side was
like a blanket pressing on us. We felt our way up the
steep street till we came to the village hall where the
dance was going on.

A cheerful young farmer took our money at the door.
We went into the hall and were caught up in a tight
mass of dancers right away. The place was packed
solid with young men in stiff, dark suits and girls in
bright dresses. They all sweated happily as they
swung and swayed to the music.

On the low platform at one end a group was
playing its heart out – piano, accordion, violin and
drums. At the other end several plump, middle-aged
women stood behind a long table, looking after the thick
ham sandwiches, home-made pies, jugs of milk and
trifles topped with cream.

Connie and I started to dance. I loved it. Without
any effort I guided Connie among the throng. I knew
dimly that we were bumping into people, but try as I
might, I could not feel my feet touching the floor. I
decided I had never been so happy in my life.

After five or six dances I felt very hungry, so Connie
and I went over to the food table. We each ate a huge
hunk of ham and egg pie. We enjoyed it so much that
we had the same again. We followed this with trifle
and then went back to dance again. It was half-way
through the next dance that my feet began to feel
strangely heavy. They began to drag. Connie felt
heavy, too. I seemed to be carrying her around.

She looked up. Her face was white. She mumbled

something about feeling odd. Then she ran for the ladies' room. A few minutes later she came out. Her face was green. She staggered over to me and said, 'I want some fresh air. Take me out-side.'

I took her out-side and it was as if I had stepped on to a ship. The ground moved up and down under my feet. I could hardly stand. Holding Connie's arm, I went to lean against the wall of the hall but this did not help as the wall, too, was moving about. I felt sick. I thought of the ham and egg pie and groaned.

'Oh, God,' I moaned, 'why did I drink all that beer?'

But I had to look after Connie. I put my arm round her and said,

'Come on, we'd better start walking.' We began to stagger round the building. We stopped every now and then while I got my breath back and shook my head to clear my brain.

But I was not steering very straight and I forgot that the village hall was on a little steep-sided hill. One moment we were walking on nothing, next we were slipping down a muddy bank. We ended up in a heap on the hard road at the bottom.

I lay there happily enough, till I heard a sad whimper from near by. Connie! I had forgotten her. When I helped her up, however, she was not hurt, and nor was I. After all the beer we had drunk we were both as limp as rag dolls when we fell.

We went back and stood just inside the door. Connie looked a sight. Her wet hair was all over her face. Tears ran slowly down her muddy face. My suit was covered in dirt and so was my face. We stood close together, leaning on each other in the door-way. My stomach was still heaving.

Then I heard somebody say good evening. It was a woman's voice. Two people stood looking at us with interest. They had just come through the door. It was

Helen and a man. She said, 'We thought we would just look in for a few moments to see how the dance was going. Are you enjoying it?'

She was smiling her kind smile but she looked strained as her eyes went from me to Connie and back again. I could not speak, but stood looking at her, seeing only her calm beauty in the crush and noise. It seemed for a moment that it would be the most natural thing in the world to throw my arms around her. Instead, I just nodded stupidly.

'Well, then, we must be off. Good night,' she said and smiled again.

The man gave me a cold nod and they went out.

39 A dog's life

It looked as if I was going to reach the road all right. I was thankful, because seven o'clock in the morning in the winter dawn was no time to be digging my car out of the snow.

It had not been snowing on my way to my early call, but the wind had been growing stronger. The top snow, blown by the wind, had started to build up into drifts.

This was how all blocked roads began. Back at the farm I had heard the wind out-side the cow-shed getting louder. I had wondered if I would win the race home.

On the way back the drifts had stopped being pretty and lay deep across the road. My little car had managed to get through them, skidding at times with wheels spinning. Now I could see the main road a few hundred yards ahead.

But just over there on the left was Cote House, where I was treating a bullock. He had eaten too many frozen turnips. I had been going to visit him later in the day, but I did not fancy coming back here if I could help it. A light in the kitchen window told me that the family was up, so I turned and drove into the yard.

There was a small porch out-side the farm-house door. The wind had driven the snow inside the porch, forming a smooth, two-foot heap across the door. As I leaned across to knock on the door, the top of the heap moved. There was something in there, something big. It was creepy standing in the half-light watching the snow parting to reveal a rough, hairy body. Some wild animal must have strayed in, looking for warmth. But it was bigger than a fox or anything else I could think of.

Just then the door opened and the light from inside streamed out. Peter Trenholm and his wife were smiling at me from the kitchen and asking me in. They were a cheerful young couple.

'What's that?' I gasped, pointing at the animal that was shaking snow from its coat. Peter grinned and told me that it was Tip, one of their dogs.

'Tip, your dog? What's he doing under a pile of snow?' I asked.

'It just blew in on him, I suppose. That's where he sleeps, just out-side the door,' Peter said.

I stared at the farmer and said, 'You mean he sleeps there, out in the open, every night?'

'Yes, always. Summer and winter. But don't look at me like that, Mr Herriot. It's his own choice. The other dogs have a warm bed in the cow-shed, but Tip won't think of it. He's fifteen now, and he's been sleeping there since he was a pup. I remember when my father was alive he tried all ways to get him to sleep inside but it was no good,' Peter said.

I looked at the old dog in surprise. He certainly did not look fifteen. It was hard to think that any animal living in these cold uplands should choose to sleep out-side and be healthy on it. I had to look hard to see any sign of his great age at all.

He shook the last snow from his coat, went up to the farmer and barked. Peter Trenholm laughed and said, as he led the way to the farm buildings, 'You see, he's ready to be off. He's a devil for his work is Tip.'

I followed, stumbling over frozen ruts, like iron under the snow. I bent my head against the knife-like wind. It was good to open the cow-shed door and escape into the warmth.

There was a mixture of animals in the long building. The dairy cows took up most of its length. Then there were a few young cows, some bullocks and the other farm dogs. They were in an empty stall, deep in straw. The cats were there too, so it must have been warm. No animal is a better judge of comfort than a cat. They could just be seen, rolled up in the straw.

Tip joined the other dogs. They were a young dog and a bitch with three half-grown pups. You could see that Tip was boss.

The bullock that I had come to see was looking a lot better. Yesterday his big first stomach had been swollen with frozen turnips. He had been sore and groaning with discomfort. But today as I put my ear against his side I could hear faint rumblings, instead of the deathly silence of yesterday. I was pleased that the stomach wash-out that I had given him seemed to have done some good. I decided to give him another today, to put him completely right.

I jammed the wooden gag in the bullock's mouth and did it up behind his horns. Then I passed the tube down into the stomach and pumped in the stomach wash. When I had finished I put my ear to his side again and listened. I could hear gurgles and rumblings even more plainly now. I smiled to myself. It had worked.

As I cleaned up my instruments I could hear the hiss of milk hitting the side of the bucket as Peter's brother got on with the morning milking. As he came down the shed with a full bucket he filled the dogs' dishes with a few pints of warm milk. Tip strolled up to drink some from his bowl. While he was drinking the young dog tried to push his way in. A snap from Tip's jaws only just missed his nose. He moved off to another dish. However, Tip did not protest when the bitch and the pups joined him at the bowl.

I went to the farm-house for a cup of tea and when I came out it was daylight. But the sky was grey and the wind bent the trees near the house almost double. It made me feel that the best place on earth was by the side of that bright fire in the farm kitchen.

Most people would have felt like that, but not old Tip. He was with Peter as he loaded a cart with some hay bales for the young cattle in the out-side barns. As Peter set off over the fields Tip jumped on to the back of the cart.

As I put my things in the boot and drove away I carried with me the picture of Tip, who did not want to know about the softer things of life and slept in the place of honour, at his master's door.

40 A nice surprise

'Could Mr Herriot see my dog, please?'

Words I had often heard, but the voice was enough to stop me in my tracks. It came from the waiting room, just as I was passing.

It couldn't be! No, of course it couldn't be. But it sounded just like Helen. On tip-toe I went up to the door and peeped through the crack. All I could see was a hand resting on the head of a sheep dog, the hem of a skirt and a pair of legs.

They were nice legs, not skinny. Suddenly a head bent over to speak to the dog. I had a close-up of the small, straight nose and the dark hair falling across the smooth cheek.

I was still looking, hardly able to believe my eyes, when Tristan shot out of the room and bumped into me. He grabbed my arm and pulled me along the passage and into the dispensary. He shut the door and whispered, 'It's her! She wants to see you! Not me or Siegfried, but you!' He looked at me for a moment, wide-eyed, and then opened the door and tried to push me into the passage.

'What the hell are you waiting for?' he hissed. 'What more do you want? Go on, get in there!'

I did not give myself any time to think. I marched straight into the waiting room. Helen looked up and smiled – just the same friendly smile as when I first met her.

We just looked at each other for some moments and then, when I didn't say anything, she looked down at the dog.

'It's Dan in trouble this time,' she said. 'He's our sheep dog but we're so fond of him. He's just like one of the family.'

The dog wagged his tail at the sound of his name, but yelped when he came towards me. I bent down and patted his head, saying, 'I see he's holding up a hind leg.'

'Yes, he jumped over a wall this morning and he's been like that ever since. I think it's something quite bad. He can't put any weight on the leg,' Helen said.

'Right, bring him through to the other room and I'll have a look at him. Take him along in front of me and I'll be able to watch how he walks,' I said, holding open the door. She went through ahead of me with the dog.

I found I was watching how Helen walked for the first few yards. It was a long passage and by the time we had reached the second bend I had managed to drag my eyes back to the dog.

He had put his hip out of joint. It had to be that, the way he carried his leg underneath his body with the paw just brushing the ground. This was a bad injury, but the chances were I could put it right – and look good at the same time.

In the operating room I lifted Dan on to the table. He stood without moving while I examined his hip. There was no doubt about it, the joint was out.

The dog looked round only twice while I was going over him. Like a lot of quiet animals, he seemed ready to trust me. I felt that if I had started to cut his head off he would not have made too much fuss.

'Nice dog,' I said. 'Seems to have a good temper, too.'

'Yes,' she said, 'I hope he hasn't hurt himself too badly.'

I told her what the trouble was. I said I thought there was a good chance that I could put the joint back, because she had not hung about for days before bringing him in.

'When will you be able to start on him?' she asked.

'Right now,' I said. 'I'll just give Tristan a shout. This is a two-man job.'

'Couldn't I help?' Helen said. 'I'd very much like to, if you wouldn't mind.'

I looked at her doubtfully and pointed out that she might not like playing tug of war with Dan in the middle, even if he was unconscious. She laughed and said that she was quite strong and very used to working with animals.

'Right,' I said. 'Slip on a spare white coat and we'll begin.'

41 Back in business

The dog did not move as I pushed the needle into his vein. Soon he was unconscious, as limp as a rag doll. I took hold of the leg and spoke across the table.

'I want you to link your hands under his thigh and try to hold him there while I pull. OK? Here we go, then.'

I kept up a steady pull on the leg with my right hand, while pushing on the hip with my left hand. Helen did her part well, leaning back against the pull. Her lips pushed forward in a pout with the effort.

I suppose there must be a foolproof way of doing this job, a method which works the very first time. I have never been able to find it. I always have to use the trial and error method. I was wondering what

Helen was thinking about this wrestling match, when I heard a quiet click. I was very glad to hear it.

'Well, that's it,' I said. 'Hope it stays put. We'll have to keep our fingers crossed. The odd one does pop out again, but I think this one will be all right.'

'Poor Dan,' Helen said. 'How long will it be before he comes round?'

'Oh, he'll be out for the rest of the day. When he starts to wake up tonight I want you to be around to steady him in case he falls and puts the thing out again. Perhaps you would give me a ring. I'd like to know how things are,' I said, picking Dan up in my arms. I was carrying him along the passage to the car, when I met Mrs Hall. She was carrying a tray with two cups.

'I was just having a cup of tea, Mr Herriot,' she said. 'I thought you and the young lady might like a cup.'

This was unusual. I looked at her. Was it possible Tristan had put her up to this? Her face told me nothing. I said, 'Thanks very much, Mrs Hall. I'll just put the dog out in the car first.'

I went out and settled Dan on the back seat of Helen's car. Helen was already drinking a cup of tea by the time I went in again. This time we could think of plenty to talk about. Maybe it was because I was on my own ground. At any rate, I found myself chatting away without any effort, just as I had done on that hill when we first met.

Mrs Hall's teapot was empty and all the biscuits eaten by the time I saw Helen off and started on my round.

Later that evening I still felt at ease when I heard her voice on the phone. 'Dan is up and walking about,' she said. 'He's still a bit wobbly but his leg seems fine.'

'Oh, great! He's got the first stage over,' I said.

There was a pause at the other end of the line, and then she said, 'Thank you so much for what you've done. We really were worried about him. We're very grateful.'

'Not at all. I'm pleased, too. He's a grand dog.' I waited for a moment. It had to be now. 'Oh, you remember we were talking about Scotland today. While I was passing the cinema this afternoon I saw they're showing a film about Scotland. I thought maybe . . . I wondered if perhaps, er . . . you might like to come and see it with me.'

Another pause and my heart did a quick thud-thud. 'All right,' Helen said. 'Yes, I'd like that. When? Friday night? Well, thank you. Good-bye till then.'

I put down the phone, my hand shaking. Why did I make such heavy weather of these things? However, it didn't matter. I was back in business.

42 Second chance

Tristan was unpacking medicine bottles. He was lifting them out of a tea-chest and stacking them in rows on shelves. When I came in, he decided it was time for a rest. He sat on the tea-chest and pulled out a packet of cigarettes. He lit one and said to me, 'You're taking her to the pictures, then?'

'Yes, that's right. In about an hour,' I said.

'Mm,' he said, giving me a funny look. 'Mm, I see.'

'Well, what are you looking like that for?' I said. 'Anything wrong with the pictures?'

'No, nothing. No, I'm sure you'll have a nice time. It's just that . . .' He scratched his head. 'I thought you might have gone in for something a bit more . . . well . . . interesting.'

I gave a bitter laugh. 'Look, remember the last time I took her out? I tried something interesting then. Oh, I'm not blaming you, Triss, but as you know it was a complete shambles. I just don't want anything to go wrong tonight. I'm playing safe.'

'Well, I won't argue with you,' said Tristan. 'You can't get much safer than the Darrowby Plaza.'

Later, as I was having a bath, I could not keep out the thought that Tristan was right. I was being a bit of a coward taking Helen to the local cinema. But there was some comfort in the thought that it was another start, even though a small one.

As I left the house I felt quite light of heart. Perhaps it was because there was just a hint of spring in the air. It was still cold, but the promise of sunshine and warm grass and milder days was there.

You could easily miss the Plaza, unless you knew where to look. It was tucked in between the chemist's and the iron-monger's. The door was not much bigger than a shop-front. The place was in darkness. I was in good time but the show was due to start in ten minutes or so and there was no sign of life.

I had not dared to tell Tristan that I had fixed it with Helen that we were to meet out-side the cinema. I had not told her I would call for her at her house. With a car like mine I could not be sure of getting anywhere on time, or indeed at all.

The black thoughts went when I saw Helen coming across the market-place. She smiled and waved cheerfully, as if being taken to the Darrowby Plaza was the biggest treat a girl could wish for. When she came up to me there was a soft flush on her cheeks and her eyes were bright.

Everything was suddenly perfect. I felt sure this was going to be a good night. Nothing was going to spoil it. After she had said, 'Hello!' she told me that her dog was running about with no trace of a limp. I felt very pleased.

The only thing that worried me was that the cinema still seemed to be shut. I looked around. There was not a queue but little groups of people were standing here and there. Nobody else seemed worried, so it must be all right.

As indeed it was. Just two minutes before the picture was due to start a man came round the corner at top speed on a bike. He came to a sudden halt out-side the cinema, jumped off his bike and opened the doors for us. He switched on the lights for us, then tore off his coat, showing us that he was in full evening dress. The manager had arrived.

While this was going on a very fat lady came from nowhere and squeezed herself into the pay-box. The show was ready to start.

We all began to go inside. The little boys put down their ninepences and punched each other as they passed through the curtain into the stalls. The rest of us went upstairs to the one-and-sixpenny seats in the balcony. The manager smiled and bowed as we passed.

We stopped at a row of pegs at the top of the stairs. Some people hung up their coats. I was surprised to see Maggie Robinson, the blacksmith's daughter, there, taking the tickets. She looked very interested when she saw us and giggled. She took our tickets and in we went.

43 Another shambles

The place was very hot. If it had not been for the smell of the old seats we might have been in the jungle. Maggie steered us through the heat to our places and as I sat down I saw that there was no arm between the two seats.

'You're in the courting seats,' said Maggie and fled, her hand to her mouth.

The lights were still on. I looked round the balcony. There were only about twelve other people dotted here and there. They sat, quiet, waiting for the film. By the side of the screen the hands of a clock stood at twenty past four.

But it was all right, sitting there with Helen, apart from the heat. I was gasping for air like a goldfish. I was just beginning to relax when a little man in front of us, sitting with his wife, turned slowly round. His old face was grim and he fixed his eyes on me in a long stare. We faced each other for some time before he spoke.

'She's dead,' he said.

I was filled with horror. 'Dead?' I said.

'Yes. Dead,' he said, still staring at me.

I swallowed a couple of times. Then I managed to say, 'I'm sorry to hear that. Very sorry.'

He nodded grimly and kept staring at me as if he wanted me to say more. Then he turned away, and settled in his seat.

I looked helplessly at his back. Who, in God's name, was this? What was he talking about? What was dead? Cow? Bitch? Sow? My mind began to race over the cases I had seen in the past week. That face did not seem to fit in anywhere.

Helen was looking at me. I managed a small smile, but the spell was gone. I started to say something to her when the little man began to turn round again.

He fixed me once again with an angry stare.

'I don't think there was anything wrong with her stomach,' he said. He turned back to the screen again.

By this time my nerves were in a state. Suddenly the lights went off which made me worse. At the same time a roar of noise blasted my ear drums. It was the news. It seemed the loud-speakers, like the heating, were very powerful and turned up full. I shut my eyes and tried to place the man in front. When the news finished I had got back about three weeks, still with no luck.

There was a moment's quiet. Then the music broke out again. This was the big film. The film about Scotland was on later. It was supposed to be a tender love story and there was a lot of kissing. This was spoiled for me because every kiss on the screen made all the little boys down-stairs make long, drawn-out sucking noises.

All the time I was getting hotter. I opened my coat wide and undid the button on my collar but I still felt a bit light-headed. The little man in front was in a big over-coat and did not seem to mind. Twice the film broke down and we stared for several minutes at a blank screen while a storm of whistles and clapping came from down-stairs.

Maggie Robinson, standing in the dim light by the curtain, seemed very interested in us. Whenever I looked up, her eyes were fixed on us with a knowing smile.

It was a relief when the last close-up came to an end and the lights went up. I was a bit worried about Helen. I had seen her mouth twitch now and again

118

as the evening wore on. Then sometimes there was a deep frown on her forehead. I wondered if she was upset. Just then Maggie arrived wearing a tray round her neck. She stood over us, smiling, while I bought two choc ices.

I had taken only one bite when the man in front turned round again. The eyes staring from that grim mask were as cold as ever.

'I knew right from the start,' he said, 'that you were on the wrong track.'

'Is that so?' I said.

'Yes. I've been among beasts for fifty years, and they never go on like that when it's in the stomach,' he said.

'Don't they?' I said. 'You're right, I expect.'

This, instead of calming him down, made him quite excited. He waved a finger at me and said, 'For one thing a beast with a bad stomach is always hard in its muck.'

'I see,' I said.

'If you think back,' he said, 'this one's muck was soft, real soft.'

'Yes, yes, quite,' I said quickly. I glanced across at Helen. This was great, just what I wanted to make her feel romantic.

He sniffed and turned away.

Once again we were plunged into darkness. The noise blasted out again. I thought: there's something wrong. What was this cowboy music? Then the title came up on the screen: *Arizona Guns*.

I turned to Helen in alarm and said, 'What's going on? This is supposed to be the Scottish film we came to see, isn't it?'

'It's supposed to be,' Helen said, smiling, 'but I'm afraid it's not going to be. They often change the second film without saying anything. Nobody seems to mind.'

I sat back in my seat. Well, I had done it again. No dance at the Reniston, wrong film tonight. I was a genius in my own way.

'I'm sorry,' I said, 'I hope you don't mind too much.'

She shook her head and said, 'Not a bit. Anyway, let's give this one a chance. It may be all right.'

But as the old cowboy film went on, I gave up hope. This was going to be another of those evenings. I watched gloomily as the gang of cowboys galloped for the fourth time past the same rock. I was not ready for the deafening shots that rang out. They made me jump.

It made the chap in the next seat to me jump too. He had been dead asleep.

'Hello! Hello! Hello!' he yelled, then jumped up and waved his arms about. He gave me a back-hander on the head and pushed me rather hard against Helen's shoulder. I began to say I was sorry when I saw that her mouth was twitching again. This time the twitch seemed to spread all over her face. She was trying hard not to laugh but she could not stop herself any longer. She lay back in her seat and laughed helplessly.

I had never seen a girl laugh like this. She lay back her head on the back of the seat, legs stretched out in front of her, arms dangling by her sides. She took her time about it and waited till she could keep her face straight again before she turned to me and said, 'Look, next time, why don't we just go for a walk?

I settled down. The chap in the seat next to me seemed to have gone off to sleep again. His snores were now almost as loud as the bangs and howls from the screen. I still had not the smallest idea who that little man in front could be. I had the feeling that he had not finished with me yet. The clock still said twenty past four. Maggie was still staring at us, and the sweat ran down my back.

The place was not all I could have wished for, but never mind. There was going to be a next time.

44 A day at the races

I could see that Siegfried had something pretty important on his mind one morning at breakfast, so I asked him what it was.

He got up from his chair and walked over to the window and looked out at the empty street.

'I was just about to ask your advice, James. It's about this letter I got this morning. Here, read it,' he said.

I read the letter and said, 'Sorry. I don't get it. It's only an invitation from somebody called Major General Ransom to go to Brawton races on Saturday. What's the problem? You like racing.'

'Ah, but it's not so simple as that,' said Siegfried. 'This is a sort of test. General Ransom is one of the big boys in horse-racing in the North-West. They are looking for a new vet to look after all the race-meetings. The job would be to deal with owners who may be using drugs to help their horses win. Well, I've been told that they think I might be the man for the job. That's why they want to see me on Saturday. The idea is to have a day at the races with me and size me up.'

'If you got the job, would you have to give up this job?' I asked. A chill wind seemed to creep around me at the idea.

'No, no, but it would mean spending something like three days a week on the race-courses. I'm wondering if that wouldn't be a bit too much.'

I told Siegfried that I didn't know enough about race-horses and I didn't like racing, so I couldn't give him any advice about the job. However, I pointed out that he loved horses and was very interested in horses and races.

'You're right, James,' he said. 'And there's no doubt the extra money would be very handy. I'll go to Brawton races on Saturday and we'll see how it turns out. You must come too.'

It was nearly noon on Saturday when I opened the front door to General Ransom. He was a short square man with a moustache. With him was a man called Colonel Tremayne, who was tall, with a hawk-nose. Both men had the air of being used to giving orders. Two women in tweeds stood behind them on the lower step. There was not a smile between the four of them.

I took them into the sitting-room and gave them some sherry as Siegfried had asked me to. He came in as I was pouring, and I nearly dropped the bottle. He looked marvellous. He had on a beautifully cut suit, and he had just shaved. He took off a brand-new hat as he came in.

The General, the Colonel and their ladies looked very impressed. The Colonel even managed to smile, but the ladies just went to pieces. Their stern faces were covered in big sloppy smiles. I felt very proud of my handsome boss.

After sherry we set off in Siegfried's Rover. Tristan had spent the morning cleaning it. I couldn't help feeling that I was the only thing about the whole party that wasn't as smart as paint.

We had lunch at the course. Siegfried looked very much at home with the smoked salmon, cold chicken and champagne. There was no doubt he was a great success. He talked about racing in a clever and interesting way with the men, and was charm itself to their wives. It was quite certain at this time that he had the job in the bag.

After lunch we went down to the paddock and had a look at the horses who were going to race first. I could see Siegfried enjoying every moment as he took in the scene. He was the picture of a man who just knew he was going to have a good day.

Merryweather, the course vet, joined us to watch the first race. Siegfried and he were chatting after the race when the 'vet wanted' sign went up. A horse had slipped at the last bend and still was not up. The three of us, Merryweather, Siegfried and I, got into Merryweather's car.

Within seconds we were racing down the course to the last bend. Merryweather said that he hoped the horse had not broken his leg, because he hated shooting horses.

It didn't look too good when we got to the spot. The horse lay still on its side. Only its ribs were moving as it breathed.

The jockey, blood pouring from a cut head, said, 'What do you think, sir? Has he broken a leg?'

Merryweather examined the horse's legs carefully.

'Nothing wrong there,' he said. Then he pointed to the horse's head. 'Look at his eyes.'

We looked. The horse's eyes flickered from side to side.

'Concussion?' Siegfried said.

'That's it. He's just had a bang on the head.' Merryweather looked much happier. When we had helped the horse to his feet Merryweather went on, 'Well, that wasn't so bad. He'll be all right after a rest.'

Siegfried started to reply when we heard somebody calling Siegfried from behind the rails. It was a stout, red-faced man. We went over to him. Siegfried looked closer at the man. He was dressed very shabbily, and looked as if he knew what hard times were.

Then Siegfried cried out in delight, 'Stewie Brannon! Here, James, come and meet an old friend of mine. We went through college together.'

I had already heard so much about Stewie Brannon from Siegfried that I felt I knew him already. Siegfried had said that Stewie was a young man who seemed most unlikely to succeed when they were at college. He hated work, and disliked washing and shaving. He was a most likable man, though, and very warm and friendly.

Siegfried called over to Merryweather, 'When you get back, will you tell my friends I've just met a very old friend? I'll only be a few minutes.'

Merryweather waved and said that he would, and drove back up the course as we ducked under the rails.

Siegfried grabbed Stewie by the arm and said, 'Come on, Stewie, where can we get a drink?'

45 All for the best

We went into the long low bar under the stand, and Siegfried began to order drinks. As the drinks kept coming Siegfried and Stewie talked and talked. I didn't butt in. I sat listening, feeling more and more happy. Stewie talked of his wife and five children and how they always found it hard to make ends meet, but were always very happy.

After what seemed a very short time we all stood up and I was surprised to find everything around me was swaying gently. When the swaying stopped I had another surprise. The big bar was almost empty.

'Stewie,' Siegfried said, 'the meeting's over. Do you know we've been sitting talking here for two hours?'

'And very nice too. Far better than giving the bookies our hard-earned money.' As Stewie got up he hung on to the table and stood blinking.

'There's one thing, though,' Siegfried said. 'I came here with a party and they must be wondering where I've got to. Tell you what, come and meet them.'

We walked back to the paddock. There was no sign of the General and his party. At last we found them in the car park, standing near the Rover. They did not look pleased. Most of the other cars had gone.

Siegfried, looking very happy indeed, said, 'I'm sorry to have left you, but a rather wonderful thing has happened. I would like you to meet my very dear friend Mr Stewart Brannon.'

Four cold faces turned to look at Stewie. His big fat face was redder than ever and he was sweating. His coat was all buttoned up wrong. It made the poor, shabby old thing look worse than ever.

The General looked grim and nodded, the Colonel looked as if he was grinding his teeth. The ladies froze and looked away.

'Yes, yes,' grunted the General. 'But we've been waiting here some time and we want to get home.'

Siegfried waved a hand and said we would leave right away. Then as he turned to Stewie to say a fond good-bye, he began to feel in his pockets for the car key. After he had gone through his pockets about five times, he stopped and thought hard. Then he began to empty his pockets on to the bonnet of the car.

It wasn't just the lost key that worried me. Siegfried had drunk a lot of whisky. He was swaying a little and his hat had slid over one eye. He kept dropping things as he pulled them from his pocket.

I had a look at the General and his friends. They had watched the search in silence. The General was the first to explode.

'Great heavens, Farnon, have you lost the key or haven't you? If the damn thing's lost, we must do something. We can't have the ladies standing around here any longer.'

There was a little cough from Stewie. He swayed forward and whispered something in Siegfried's ear. Siegfried shook his hand.

'By God, Stewie, that's kind of you!' He turned to us and said, 'There's nothing to worry about. Mr Brannon has said he will take us home. He's gone to get his car.' He pointed to Stewie, who was by then trying to make his way unsteadily through the gate of the car park.

After a while, Stewie came back and we saw a look of rage cross the General's face.

The car was a tiny Austin Seven. It must have been one of the earliest models. The paint-work was rusted and the windows were cracked. It had a hood that was tied on with bits of string.

Stewie got out, opened the door and waved us towards a pile of sacks which lay on the bare boards where the seats should have been.

'Dammit, is this supposed to be a joke?' The General's face was brick red and the veins in his neck stood out.

Just then there was a sudden roar from the Rover's engine. Siegfried had found his key at last, and had started it up.

The ladies took their seats in the back.

'Get over! I'll drive!' the General barked at Siegfried, as if he was talking to a young soldier who had done something wrong.

A couple of weeks later, as Siegfried was reading the newspaper at the breakfast table, he called out to me.

'Ah, I see Herbert Jarvis has got the job of vet for the race-courses in the North-West. Nice chap, I know him. Just the man for the job.'

I looked across at my boss to see if there was any sign that he was sad that someone else had got the job. But he didn't look at all sad.

Siegfried sighed happily. 'You know, James, everything happens for the best. Old Stewie was sent from heaven. I was never meant to get that job. I would have been as miserable as hell if I had got it. Come on, lad, let's get off into our hills and dales.'

contents

Date With Disaster!

KATE

How old? 13
Lives: in Aylesbury, with her mum, dad and sister Rachel
Favourite music: Kelis, Usher, Beyoncé, Jamelia, Joss Stone
Likes: singing, reading magazines, watching films
Wants to be: a famous singer

JOE

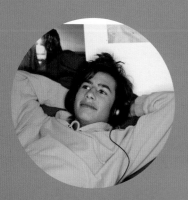

How old? 14
Lives: in Aylesbury, with his mum, dad and two brothers
Favourite music: everything from 50 Cent to Maroon 5
Likes: music, football, going to clubs, new friends
Wants to be: in a famous band, or maybe a DJ

IAN

How old? 13
Lives: in Aylesbury, with his mum and dad
Favourite music: Robbie Williams, Dido
Likes: maths, going to the cinema, playing football
Wants to be: good at lots of different things

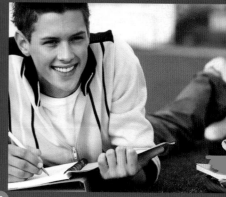

Date With Disaster!

Claire Powell

LEVEL 1

MSCHOLASTIC

Material written by: Claire Powell

Commissioning Editor: Jacquie Bloese

Editor: Fiona Beddall

Cover design: Ian Butterworth, Emily Spencer

Designer: Dawn Wilson

Illustrator: Susannah Fishburne

Picture research: Emma Bree

Photo credits: Cover: A. Pollok/Taxi/Getty Images; Rubberball; Stockdisc. **Pages 4 & 5:** Pollok/Taxi/Getty Images; Rubberball; Stockdisc; R. Stainforth/Alamy; Brand X. **Page 28:** Image100. **Pages 24 & 25:** Stockbyte; Imagesource; Hemera; S. Botterill/Getty Images; S. Bond/Alamy.

The publishers would like to acknowledge the following teachers for reporting on the manuscript:

Carine Chaput, Collège Ozar Hatorah, Toulouse, France

Kleio Drosou, Vytina High School, Arcadia, Greece

Beata Eigner, GRG, Vienna, Austria

Marie-Christine Jacquot, Collège Saint-Maimboeuf, Montbeliard, France

Adele James, Nea Paideia, Hydrari, Greece

Brigitte Neustifter, SHS Weiz, Weiz, Austria

Gertraud Noeth, Christian-von-Bomhard Schule, Uffenheim, Germany

Theodora Papavasiliou, English Language Centre, Trikala, Greece

Monique Peubez, Institution des Chartreux, Lyon, France

Maria Santoliquido, IPSCP 'Marcello Dudovich', Milan, Italy

Mary Glasgow Magazines (Scholastic Inc.)
Commonwealth House
1–19 New Oxford Street
London WC1A 1NU

Printed in Italy.

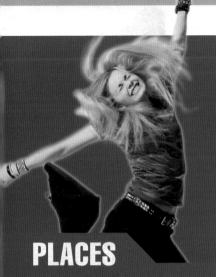

RACHEL

How old? 18
Lives: in Brighton, and with her family in Aylesbury in the holidays
Favourite music: Alicia Keys, Blue, Maroon 5
Likes: shopping, going to clubs, listening to music
Wants to be: a writer for a fashion magazine

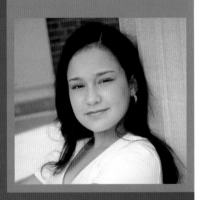

PLACES

Aylesbury: a town in England, about one hour from Oxford and London
Aylesbury Grammar and Grange School: two schools for boys and girls from 11 to 18 years old
New Look: a clothes shop in the High Street; there are lots of other shops in the High Street too
MegaSounds: a small music shop in the High Street

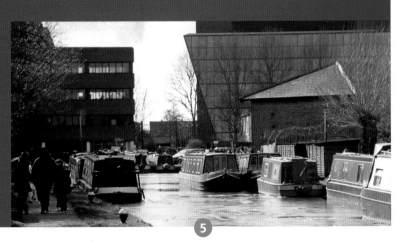

Date With

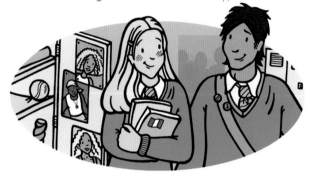

'The pictures on your locker are cool. Are you a music fan?' Kate looked up. It was the good-looking new boy from Year 9.

Kate was embarrassed. Was her face red? She smiled and hoped there was no food between her teeth from lunch. Then she said, 'Yes, I love music. I want to be a singer one day. My name's Kate. What's your name?'

'I'm Joe and I'm new here. I want to start a band. I play the guitar. Maybe you can be the singer.'

'Wow!' thought Kate. Joe was gorgeous, with his big smile and brown hair. She started to answer, but …

'Joe!' It was Sally and Melissa, two girls from Year 9. Sally had a CD in her hand. 'Joe, thanks for the CD. Are you coming to French with us?'

The two girls took Joe's arms. Joe looked at Kate and said, 'Here, listen to the new 50 Cent CD. See you!'

Kate took the CD. 'Thanks! Have fun in French!'

Disaster!

***

'Hi Kate!' It was Rachel, Kate's 18-year-old sister. Rachel was a student in Brighton, but this week she was at home on holiday. Kate was 13 and she liked the idea of her sister's life in Brighton. No mum or dad, no homework and lots of exciting student parties – fantastic!

Rachel had some photos from Brighton.

'Look. That's my new boyfriend, Sam,' said Rachel.

'Ooh, he's gorgeous,' said Kate. Kate was very pretty, with long blonde hair and big brown eyes. But she didn't have a boyfriend. For a minute, she wanted to be Rachel. Why did Rachel always have a gorgeous boyfriend, and Kate never had anyone? Then she remembered Joe.

'There's a new boy in Year 9,' she told Rachel. 'His locker's opposite mine. Lovely!'

'What, the locker or the boy?' said Rachel.

'The boy, of course!' said Kate. Her sister was very stupid sometimes. 'His name's Joe.'

***

'Kate! It's homework time!' It was Kate's mum.

'She can't do any homework today, Mum. She's thinking about Gorgeous Joe!' said Rachel.

'Please keep quiet, Rachel. Just leave me alone,' said Kate.

Kate went up to her room and sat at her desk. She looked at her maths homework. It was very difficult.

'Maybe Ian can help,' she thought. Kate sat next to Ian in maths this year, and he helped her with the difficult questions. Last week he gave her his mobile number. 'Phone me. We can do our homework together one day,' he said. Ian was nice, and good-looking too. She liked him a lot – but then she started thinking about Joe again …

***

Next day, Kate had a singing lesson at lunchtime and she didn't see Joe or Ian. At the end of the day, she walked to the bus stop with her friends. Suddenly, she remembered something.

'Oh no! My books for tonight's homework are still in my locker. I'm going back for them. See you tomorrow.'

She ran into the school and got her books. Then she saw Joe alone in a classroom. She went in.

'Joe! What are you doing here?' asked Kate.

'I've got detention,' said Joe.

'Oh no, what did you do?' Kate hated detentions.

'Well, I went to Oxford with some friends last night. We saw the Red Hot Chili Peppers there and I came home late. This morning I was tired. In English, I closed my eyes just for a minute, and the teacher saw me. He was very angry.'

Kate loved the Red Hot Chili Peppers.

'You're lucky!' said Kate. 'I wanted to go, but tickets were very expensive …'

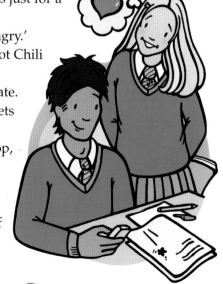

'I work at a music shop, MegaSounds, on Saturdays. Someone at the shop gave me tickets,' said Joe. 'Lots of good bands come to

Oxford. Next time, do you want to come too?'

'OK,' said Kate. 'Here's my mobile number. Text me.'

Joe smiled. 'Cool.' Then he looked at the clock. 'Oh no, it's ten past four already. I have to write 'I must not sleep in class' 300 times before five o'clock.'

Kate laughed. 'OK, see you tomorrow. And don't close your eyes again!'

chapter 2 BOYS, bOYS, bOYS ...

It was Friday lunchtime. Kate usually had her lunch in the school café with her friends. Between her classroom and the café was the football field. On her way to the café, she saw Joe on the field. She wasn't usually a football fan, but today she watched. Joe looked great in his blue and white football clothes.

'My life is boring now,' thought Kate. 'But maybe I can be Joe's girlfriend and the singer in his band. Then I can have an exciting life.'

'Hey, Kate! You don't often watch football.' It was Ian. He was in the same team as Joe. 'What do you think of the team?' he asked. 'Are we going to be better than Grange School this year?'

Some of the boys stopped and looked at Kate. Joe saw her too. She was very embarrassed. She didn't know anything about football – all her friends knew that.

'Oh, I – er – I'm late for a singing lesson! Bye!' Kate said.

'But it's Friday! You have your singing lesson after maths on Thursday!' said Ian.

'It's different this week. See you!' Kate said. Was her face red?

'That was terrible!' she thought. 'Does Joe think I'm stupid now?'

The next morning was Saturday. Kate was in bed. On Saturdays, she had breakfast in bed and read her favourite magazine, GOSSIP. She loved reading about rich and famous people and their exciting lives. 'One day I'm going to be famous too,' she thought.

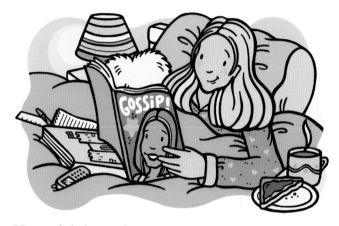

Her mobile buzzed.

'Maybe it's Joe!'

Kate looked at the phone. It was Ian. 'Why doesn't Joe call?' she thought.

'Hi, Kate! How are you?' said Ian. 'Do you want to come to my house this afternoon? We can do that maths homework together.'

A Saturday afternoon of maths! That wasn't very exciting. But their teacher wanted the homework on Monday morning.

'Yeah, OK,' said Kate. 'About four o'clock?'

'Great!' said Ian. He gave her his address. 'See you at four.'

'Hmmm,' thought Kate. 'Ian's not very cool, but he is a good friend. And I don't know very much about Joe. Is he a nice person, or is he just cool?'

She got some paper and started to write. Which boy did she like best, Ian or Joe?

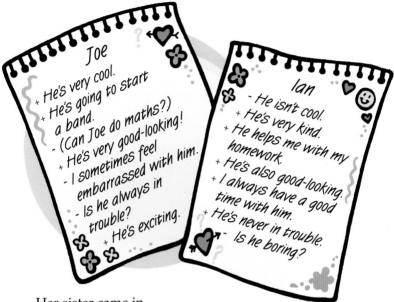

Joe
+ He's very cool.
+ He's going to start a band.
- (Can Joe do maths?)
+ He's very good-looking!
- I sometimes feel embarrassed with him.
- Is he always in trouble?
+ He's exciting.

Ian
- He isn't cool.
+ He's very kind.
+ He helps me with my homework.
+ He's also good-looking.
+ I always have a good time with him.
+ He's never in trouble.
- Is he boring?

Her sister came in.

'What's this? A letter?' she said.

Kate said, 'Don't read it! It's nothing!'

'OK, OK!' said Rachel. 'I'm going to buy some new clothes. Do you want to come?'

Kate liked shopping with Rachel. Then she had an idea. 'I want to buy some new music. Can we go to MegaSounds?' she asked.

'But we always go to HMV for CDs,' said Rachel. 'Why do you want to go to MegaSounds? Is that gorgeous new boy going to be there?'

'No,' Kate said. Well, that wasn't true. But how did her sister always know everything? And anyway, maybe Joe wasn't there today. Maybe he didn't work *every* Saturday.

chapter 3 I'm going to sell my sister!

'Do you like this T-shirt?' asked Rachel.

Rachel and Kate were at New Look in the High Street. There were a lot of clothes shops in Aylesbury, but New Look was Kate and Rachel's favourite shop.

'Yes, it's nice … But when are we going to the music shop?' asked Kate.

'Keep your hair on! The shops close at five-thirty. We've still got two hours,' said Rachel.

'Yeah, but I'm going to Ian's house at four,' said Kate.

'OK, OK. Go to the music shop. But I'm going to buy this T-shirt first. We can meet at MegaSounds,' said Rachel.

***

At MegaSounds, Kate found Joe with lots of Maroon 5 CDs in his arms. He saw her and smiled.

'Hi Kate! This is a surprise!' he said.

'Oh, hi Joe,' said Kate. 'I'm looking for the new Kelis CD.'

'Cool. She's got a great voice.' He put down the CDs in his arms and found a different one. 'Here it is,' said Joe. He gave the CD to Kate.

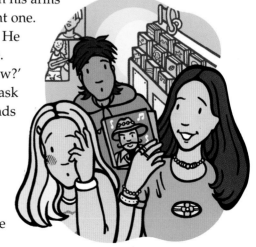

'What do I say now?' thought Kate. 'Do I ask about tickets for bands in Oxford?'

'Kate!'

It was Rachel. She had a CD in her hand.

'It's your favourite

band! Clive and the Cowboys!'

Kate and Joe looked at the CD. The singers were about 60 years old.

'Your favourite band?!' said Joe.

Kate was embarrassed. Her face was red.

'I'm going to find some more Clive music for you,' said Rachel. She walked back to the worst CDs in the shop.

'Is that your sister? She's funny,' said Joe.

Kate didn't agree. Rachel wasn't funny – she was stupid. 'I'm going to sell my sister one day!' she thought.

'Kate, I'm going to a party at Grange School tonight. Do you want to come? Clive and the Cowboys aren't going to be there, but some good DJs are playing at it.' Joe smiled at Kate. He had a gorgeous smile and beautiful big brown eyes.

'Great!' said Kate. 'And please don't listen to my sister. I'm not a big fan of Clive and the Cowboys.'

'It's OK – I didn't believe her,' said Joe. 'Anyway, a friend gave me some tickets and …'

'I'm out of here.' It was Rachel. Again. 'I want to look for a skirt in the same colour as my new T-shirt. Don't forget your maths lesson at four o'clock!'

Kate and Joe both looked at their watches. Oh no! It was ten to four already. But Kate didn't want to go. She wanted to ask Joe more about the party. Was this a date? Or did Joe have tickets for lots of friends?

'Maths on a Saturday?' Joe said. 'Oh well, don't be late. See you at the party, maybe.'

Sadly, Kate left the shop.

Her mobile buzzed. It was a message from Ian.

'WHERE R U? I'VE GOT A SURPRISE 4 U'

'A surprise for me!' thought Kate. 'Something nice, I hope.'

Chapter 4
Spots + messages + maths homework = HELP!

Kate walked to Ian's house. Ian opened the door.

His mum was in the kitchen. 'It's nice to meet you, Kate,' she said.

Ian and Kate sat at the table in the dining room. Kate opened her bag. There was a message on her mobile.

It was her sister.

'HOW'S THE DATE WITH MR MATHS?'

'Arrgh!' thought Kate. 'Rachel never stops! Ian and I aren't dating, and Rachel knows that.' Kate quickly put her phone back in her bag.

***

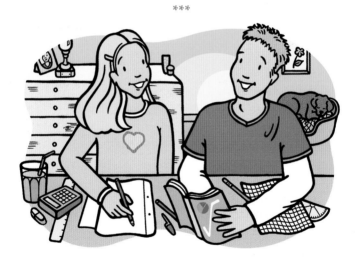

Ian was busy with the homework. He looked up at Kate and smiled. His eyes were lovely – blue, like his jeans.

'Wake up, Kate! Homework time!' he said.

'OK, but first tell me. What's the surprise?' asked Kate.

'No, I'm not going to tell you yet. Finish the homework first!' said Ian.

'Oh, tell me now! Please!' said Kate.

'OK, OK! Well, you know that new film with Orlando Bloom?' said Ian.

'Yes,' said Kate. She loved Orlando Bloom.

'The film's on at the Odeon, tonight at 6.30. I've got two tickets, so we can go together.'

'Great!' Kate smiled at Ian.

Ian was very happy. 'Fantastic! It's a date!'

Kate's smile disappeared. Maybe this wasn't a good idea. Did Ian want to be her boyfriend? What about Joe and the party tonight?

'I can't think about this now,' she thought. 'OK then, Ian,' she said. 'Let's do this homework.'

***

It was five o'clock. There was still a lot of homework.

'I can't think about maths,' thought Kate. 'I need to think about tonight. I'm going to the cinema with Ian but Joe's got a ticket for me for the party too! What am I going to do?'

Kate went to the bathroom. In the mirror, she saw a big spot on her nose.

'Oh no! Joe isn't going to want a girlfriend with a spot!' she thought. 'What can I do?! Maybe Ian has something for spots.' She looked around the bathroom, but she didn't find anything. Then she remembered – her sister sometimes used toothpaste for spots! She put some toothpaste on her nose.

In the dining room, Kate sat down quickly. She looked at her books. Ian didn't see her nose.

'There's a message on your mobile again,' said Ian.

'Oh, is there?' Kate quickly got her mobile out of her bag.

'MEET AT THE PARTY AT 8? IT'S GOING 2 B FUN.'

It was Joe. Kate was embarrassed. Did Ian see the message? She wanted to answer Joe's text – but she was next to Ian!

'Ian, sorry. I need to go to the bathroom again!'

Ian looked up. 'Are you OK, Kate? What's that on your nose?'

'Yeah, I'm OK! And my nose is OK too!' Kate ran to the bathroom. She closed the door and wrote a text to Joe.

'C U AT GRANGE SCHOOL AT 8.'

She pressed 'send'. But nothing happened! 'Oh no!' thought Kate. 'No credit! My mobile needs more credit, and I didn't buy any in town. What can I do now? I can't send a message to Joe on Ian's phone! But is Joe going to be at the party tonight anyway? Or is he going to wait at home for an answer from me?'

***

'Ian, I must go!' Kate ran into the dining room.

'But there's still lots of homework … and we can walk to the cinema together from here,' said Ian.

'I need to buy some new clothes!' said Kate.

'Keep your hair on! You don't need new clothes for the cinema. You look great now,' said Ian.

Kate thought quickly. She said, 'My sister's going back to Brighton tonight. The clothes are for her. I must go! See you!'

Ian sat in the dining room. He was very surprised. Was something wrong with Kate today?

chapter 5 Mobile mistake

Kate went up to her bedroom. She wanted to think. 'I need to text Joe, but I don't have any credit for my mobile. What can I do?' Then she had an idea.

Rachel's bedroom was empty. Rachel was in the bathroom. Kate wrote to Joe on her sister's mobile.

'THIS IS MY SISTER'S PHONE. NO CREDIT ON MINE. C U AT GRANGE SCHOOL PARTY AT 8. KATE XX'

Then she wrote Joe's number on Rachel's phone.

'What are you doing? That's my phone!' It was Rachel.

Rachel took her phone and read the message. 'You're writing love messages on my phone!' she said angrily.

'I'm sorry, but I can't use my phone. I haven't got any credit,' said Kate. 'Please can I send the message?'

'No! Don't take my things!' said Rachel.

'Rachel, please! This message is important!' said Kate.

Rachel was still angry, but she gave the phone to Kate. Kate quickly pressed 'send'.

'Next time, ask me first,' said Rachel.

After two minutes, Rachel came into Kate's room. 'There's a message for you on my phone,' she said.

Kate took the phone. It was a text from Ian.

'WHAT, NO CINEMA? BUT A PARTY IS OK 2. IAN XX'

'Oh no! I sent the message about the party to Ian,

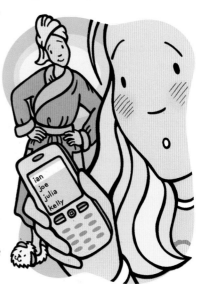

not to Joe!' Kate looked at the address book on her phone. Ian's number was next to Joe's.

'What am I going to do now? I can't go on a date with Joe and Ian to the same party!'

'Rachel, can I send another text?' asked Kate.

'Is it very important?' asked Rachel.

'Yes!' said Kate.

'OK,' said Rachel.

Kate sent a text to Ian.

'GOT A HEADACHE. STAYING AT HOME. SORRY. KATE XX'

Then she wrote to Joe.

'C U AT GRANGE SCHOOL PARTY AT 8.'

This time, she wrote Joe's number very carefully. Then she pressed 'send' and gave the phone back to her sister.

***

It was quarter to eight. Kate dressed in her favourite clothes and looked in the mirror. 'Oh no! What can I do about that terrible spot on my nose?!' she thought. But there was no time. She ran to the door.

'I'm meeting a friend from school! Bye!' said Kate to her mum and dad. They were in the living room. They always watched a film on TV on Saturday nights.

'OK! Be home before 10!' they said. Kate was lucky. Her family lived in the centre of town. It was an easy walk to the shops and cafés … and to Grange School.

Kate walked down the street to the party. 'Is Ian going to be angry with me?' she thought. 'I hope not. He doesn't need to know about my date with Joe.'

She was happy. 'Tonight's going to be fun,' she thought.

***

Kate was on the street in front of Grange School. She looked at her watch. '8.05,' she thought. 'So where's Joe?'

She looked across the street to the school door. Then she stopped.

Ian and Joe were both there!

'Oh no!' Kate went behind a tree. 'What are they doing? Why is Ian here? Does Ian know about my date with Joe? Ian mustn't see me! My text message to him said, 'Got a headache – staying at home.' What can I do?'

There was only one answer. She went home. 'This is a disaster,' she thought. 'What can I say to Ian and Joe?'

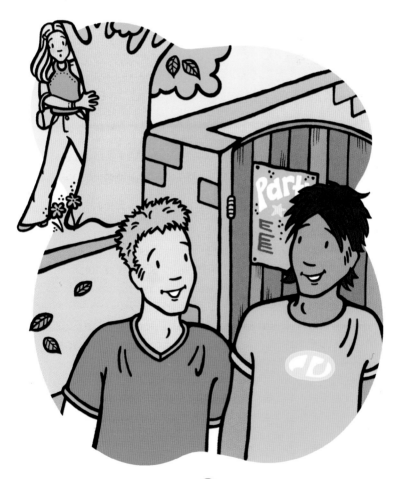

Chapter 6 Date With disaster!

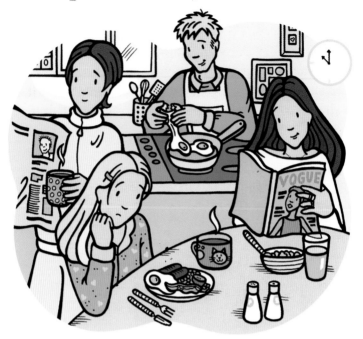

'Kate, eat your breakfast. It's going to be cold soon!' said Kate's dad. Usually Kate loved her dad's big Sunday breakfast, but today she wasn't hungry.

'Poor Kate's tired! She had two dates last night!' said Rachel.

'Is that true, Kate?' asked their mum.

'It's not true! I don't have a boyfriend!' Kate said. She ran up to her room.

Soon there was someone at her bedroom door.

'It's me – Rachel. Are you OK, Kate?' she asked.

Kate told her sister everything.

'Kate, it's OK. Ian and Joe are your friends,' said Rachel.

'Maybe,' said Kate. 'I just don't know …'

***

Kate went back to the kitchen. She heard the phone. Was it Joe or Ian? Kate didn't want to answer it.

'Hi Kate! How are you feeling?' It was Ian.

'I'm better today, thanks. And Ian, I'm very sorry about last night.'

'That's OK,' said Ian. 'I didn't see your second message at home. My mobile was in my bag and I didn't hear it. I went to Grange School and waited for you. You didn't come, so then I looked at my messages. But I met Joe at the school – you know, the new boy in Year 9, the one in my football team. Well, he had some tickets so I went to the party anyway. It was fun. I changed the tickets for the cinema. Do you want to see the film tonight? It starts at six.'

'OK, great!' said Kate. 'Let's meet at the cinema.'

They said goodbye. Kate put down the phone and thought, 'Ian isn't angry about last night, so Joe didn't talk to Ian about me. Maybe *this* date isn't going to be a disaster!'

***

'That was a great film,' said Kate. She and Ian walked out of the cinema together.

'Yes, it was good,' said Ian. 'I'm hungry now. Let's get some food.'

There was a café near the cinema. People often went there after a film. They started to walk to it.

Suddenly, Ian pointed to someone. 'Look, Kate, it's Joe!'

'OH NO!' thought Kate. 'I'm here with Ian! What's Joe going to think? I can't run away! Is this a date with disaster again?!'

It was too late. 'Joe!' shouted Ian. Joe looked up and crossed the road. Then Kate saw a girl behind Joe.

'Ian, who's that girl?' she asked.

'It's Joe's girlfriend, Laura. I met her last night at the party,' said Ian.

Kate was angry for a minute. Then she was embarrassed. 'So Joe didn't ask me on a date to the party!' she thought. 'It was just a night out with some friends! I'm so stupid.'

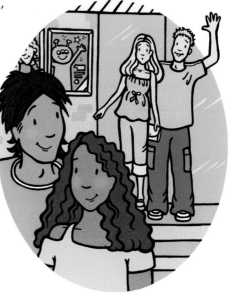

Joe was in front of them now. He smiled and said, 'Hi again, Kate. I met Ian at the party last night. Why weren't you there too?'

Kate was embarrassed. 'I had a headache.'

Then Joe said, 'Kate, this is my girlfriend, Laura. She goes to my old school in Oxford.'

'Hi,' said Kate. Was her face red? She still liked Joe, and she wasn't very happy about Laura. 'Are you going to be in Joe's band?'

'Laura plays the drums. She's fantastic,' Joe said. He smiled at Laura.

'Luckily Oxford's not very far away. I can come and play in the band here every weekend,' said Laura.

'But we still need a good singer,' said Joe. 'Kate?'

'But –' Kate didn't know. Laura had a nice smile, like Joe. 'But three isn't always a good number,' she thought. 'Can we all be friends in a band together?'

'Well, think about it,' said Joe. 'We're going to have auditions next week.'

'I can play the guitar,' said Ian suddenly. 'Can I come to the auditions too?'

Kate was surprised. She knew Ian was good at maths. But the guitar too?

Joe smiled. 'That's great, Ian. So we've got Kate the singer, Laura on the drums, Ian and me on guitar – we've got a band already! When are we going to be on MTV?!'

They all laughed.

Kate was happy now. 'I feel very lucky,' she thought. 'Joe and Ian are still my friends, and maybe I can be in a fantastic band! I don't need to be Joe's girlfriend. Friends are more important than boyfriends anyway.'

Joe and Laura went into the café. Ian waited for Kate at the café door.

'Come on, Kate! You're always dreaming!' Ian smiled.

Kate thought, 'I want to know more about Ian. He's different from Joe, but maybe he's cool too. Maybe I *can* have a boyfriend with a guitar …'

She followed her friends into the café. 'Let's talk music!' she said.

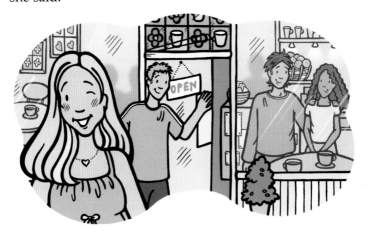

FIRST DATE

**Where do British teenagers go for their first date?
We asked some teenagers in London.**

Carly, 14 'On my first date, I went to the cinema. It's a great place for a first date, because you can talk about the film at the end!'

Paul, 12 'The best thing for a first date? A football match. My favourite team is Arsenal. I want an Arsenal fan as a girlfriend, so we can go to matches together.'

Jenny, 14 'I'd like a first date in a restaurant. Pizza's my favourite food. A restaurant is a good place because you can talk a lot. You can't talk in a cinema!'

Sam, 13 'I went to the funfair for my first date with my girlfriend. We went on lots of different rides and laughed a lot.'

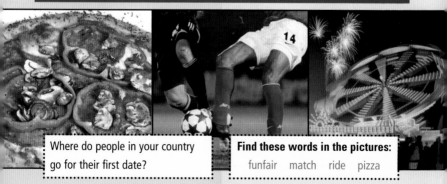

Where do people in your country go for their first date?

Find these words in the pictures:
funfair   match   ride   pizza

24

I was SO embarrassed!

It's your first date. You want to have a fantastic time, but sometimes plans go wrong …

'I had a date with a boy from my class. He asked me to the cinema. It was our first date. At the cinema, I waited and waited. It started to rain. Then he called me on my mobile. "Where are you? The film starts in two minutes!" he said. I was at the wrong cinema!' **Laura, 12**

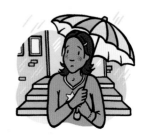

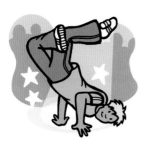

'I was at a friend's party and my new girlfriend, Anna, was with me. There was some cool music and I started to dance in the centre of the room. I did some breakdancing. Everyone watched. Suddenly, my shoe came off my foot and hit Anna on the nose! It was terrible!' **Joel, 13**

'On my first date, I went shopping with my boyfriend, Jake. We walked around the shopping centre and had a burger. Everything was cool. We saw one of my friends and I talked to her for a few minutes. Jake didn't stay with us. My friend went, and I saw Jake at the jewellery shop window. "That's nice," I thought. "He's buying me something." I walked to the window and put my arms around him. But it wasn't Jake! I didn't know this boy at all! Jake was in a shop opposite the jewellery shop and he saw everything. He laughed, but I was very embarrassed!' **Molly, 13**

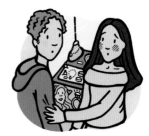

Which of these first date disasters is the worst?

Find these words in the pictures:
breakdancing   jewellery

Are you a dating

Do you have dating disasters like Kate? Or are you good at the dating game? Answer the questions and find out.

1 There's a new boy/girl in your class. You like him/her a lot. What do you say?

☐ **a.** 'Hello, my name's … . What are your hobbies?'

☐ **b.** 'Hi. You're the best-looking person in our class. Come out with me on Saturday.'

☐ **c.** Nothing. You're too embarrassed.

2 You're on the bus. A gorgeous boy/girl phones you on your mobile. What do you do?

☐ **a.** Have a short conversation and plan to meet at the weekend.

☐ **b.** Talk loudly for an hour on the bus. Some people on the bus look at you angrily. You don't care – this is true love!

☐ **c.** Plan a conversation in your head, then answer. But it's too late. The person at the other end didn't wait.

3 It's your first date, and you like this boy/girl a lot. Five minutes before the date, he/she phones you and says, 'I'm sorry. I'm going to be late.' What do you do?

☐ **a.** Ask, 'Are you very busy? Do you want to meet on a different day?'

☐ **b.** Feel angry and say, 'I don't wait for anyone! Enjoy your next date – with a new boy/girlfriend!'

☐ **c.** Say nothing and start to cry.

disaster?

4 **You're meeting your new boy/girlfriend for a pizza. What do you wear?**

☐ **a.** Your favourite jeans and a cool T-shirt.

☐ **b.** Expensive new clothes. You look like Orlando Bloom/Keira Knightley at the Oscars.

☐ **c.** You can't decide. In the end, you wear the same things as yesterday. They're a bit dirty, but who cares?

5 **You've got a date. At home, your parents ask, 'Are you going to meet your new boy/girlfriend?' What do you say?**

☐ **a.** 'I'm meeting someone from school. He/she's nice, but we're just friends.' You don't feel embarrassed.

☐ **b.** 'Yes, I'm meeting (name) and he/she's the love of my life!'

☐ **c.** 'I'm not meeting anyone. I'm just taking the dog for a walk.' You feel very embarrassed.

Which answer did you give most?

a. Fantastic! You're very good at the dating game. You make friends with a boy/girl first and think about love second.

b. You love dreaming about love, but sometimes this isn't a good idea. Life isn't always like a dream. Try to think about boys/girls as friends too.

c. Maybe you like someone a lot. But is it difficult to talk to him/her? Many people have the same trouble. Can you go out with him/her with a group of your friends? Sometimes this is easier than a date for two.

MOBILE

Text messages are cheap, quick and easy! With a text, you can:

▸▸ say a quick hello
▸▸ send pictures and funny stories
▸▸ plan a day out with your friends

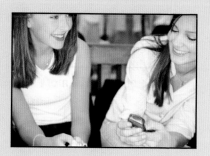

And it's fun too. Use these abbreviations and write the best texts in town!

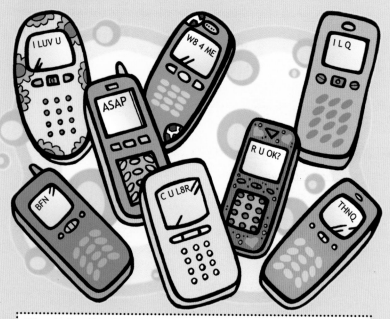

What do the abbreviations mean? For some help, look below.

bye for now	I like you	as soon as possible	I love you
see you later	wait for me	thank you	are you OK?

MAD

DID YOU KNOW?

▸▸ In the UK, teenagers send over 1 billion text messages every month. That's more than 30 million texts a day!

▸▸ What do 70% of American teenagers want for Christmas? Mobile phones!

▸▸ In the UK, 90% of people from 11 to 16 years old have mobile phones. 10% of them talk on their mobiles for more than 45 minutes a day.

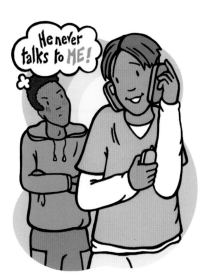

Are you mobile mad? Answer the questions and find out.

a) Do you always want a smaller mobile phone?   Yes / No

b) Your friend's got a new mobile. He/she can take photos and use the internet with it. Do you want one too?   Yes / No

c) You are bored. Do you play a game on your phone?   Yes / No

d) You leave your mobile at home. You live 20 minutes away. Do you go home and get your phone?   Yes / No

e) Do you use your phone more than five times a day?   Yes / No

You get a point for every 'yes' answer.

4 – 5 points: You can't live without your mobile phone!

2 – 3 points: You like having a mobile, but you don't use it all the time.

0 – 1 points: Mobile phones aren't very important to you. You like talking to your friends face to face.

chapters 1–2

Before you read

1 What is the past simple of these irregular verbs?
   a) see **b)** sit **c)** take **d)** tell **e)** think **f)** give **g)** run
   h) know **i)** get

2 Which of these adjectives describe:
   a) personality **b)** appearance **c)** feelings?
   You can use your dictionary.
   gorgeous   **good-looking**   **cool**
   pretty   **angry**   **stupid**   **embarrassed**

3 Which of these words isn't something about school? Use
   your dictionary.
   a) detention **b)** homework **c)** classroom **d)** fan
   e) locker **f)** lesson **g)** maths

4 Complete the sentences with these verbs.
   text   **smile**   **buzz**   **laugh**
   a) Did my mobile … ? Oh good, I've got a message.
   b) I always … very loudly at funny stories.
   c) I've got my mobile, so he can … me his address.
   d) … for the camera, please.

After you read

5 Answer the questions.
   a) Kate meets Joe at the lockers. Do they talk about:
      i) homework ii) music iii) films?
   b) How does Kate know Ian?
   c) Why does Joe have a detention after school?
   d) Does Kate often watch football?
   e) Where do Rachel and Kate want to go on Saturday
      afternoon?

6 What do you think?
   a) Would you like a sister like Rachel? Why/Why not?
   b) Who is a better boyfriend for Kate, Ian or Joe? Why?

chapters 3–4

Before you read

7 Answer the questions. You can use your dictionary.

a) Your mobile hasn't got any credit. Can you call someone on it?

b) You have a big spot on your face. Do you feel gorgeous?

c) Which place is better for a date: a bank or a party?

d) You look in a mirror. What can you see?

8 Complete the sentences with these words. You can use your dictionary.

ticket   press   toothpaste   send

a) You can't get on the train without a … .

b) I clean my teeth with white … .

c) I … letters to people in lots of different countries.

d) Oh no! I did my homework on the computer but I didn't … 'save'. Now I can't find it.

After you read

9 Are these sentences true or false? Correct the false sentences.

a) Kate sees Ian at the music shop.

b) Rachel finds a CD for Kate. It's Kate's favourite music.

c) Joe wants to go to the party with Kate on Saturday evening.

d) Ian helps Kate with her English homework.

e) Ian has got tickets for the cinema.

f) Kate puts toothpaste on her nose because she has a spot.

g) Kate can't send a message to Joe because she has no credit on her phone.

h) Kate walks to the cinema with Ian.

10 What do you think?

a) Is Kate going to go to the cinema with Ian? What about the party with Joe?

b) Two people are going to enjoy the evening. One person is not. Who's going to have a bad time: Joe, Ian or Kate?

chapters 5-6

Before you read

11 Match these words with the correct definitions.

a) Take an aspirin for that ...
b) I wanted to be in the film, so I decided to go to the ...
c) Everything went wrong. It was a ...
d) I love being loud, so I'm learning to play the ...

i) drums.
ii) disaster.
iii) headache.
iv) audition.

12 Is Kate going to have a boyfriend at the end of the story? Who?

After you read

13 Kate needs to send a message to Joe. Answer the questions.
a) How does Kate send a text about the party?
b) Why is Rachel angry?
c) Who gets Kate's message about the party?

14 Are these sentences true or false? Correct the false sentences.
a) Kate sent the text about the party to Ian by mistake.
b) Joe and Ian were both at the party.
c) Kate went to the party and danced a lot.
d) The next day, Joe and Kate went to the cinema together.
e) Laura was at the party on Saturday.
f) Ian plays the drums.
g) Kate likes Ian a lot at the end of the story.

15 What do you think?
a) Is Laura lucky? Is Joe a good boyfriend? Why/Why not?
b) What's going to happen to Kate, Ian, Laura and Joe? Think about:
i) their love life   ii) Joe's band